29.95

NCLEX-RN®
6 Comprehensive Tests

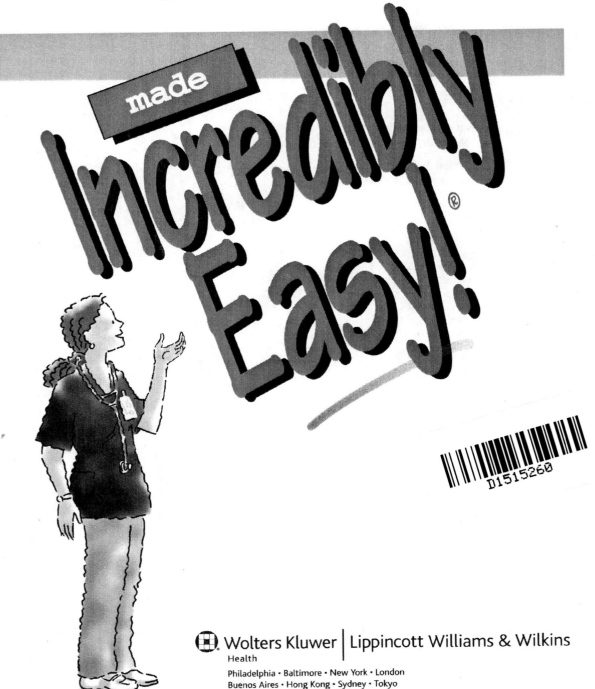

made
Incredibly
Easy!®

⊞. Wolters Kluwer | Lippincott Williams & Wilkins
Health

Philadelphia · Baltimore · New York · London
Buenos Aires · Hong Kong · Sydney · Tokyo

Staff

Publisher
Chris Burghardt

Clinical Director
Joan M. Robinson, RN, MSN

Clinical Project Manager
Beverly Ann Tscheschlog, RN, MS

Clinical Editor
Jennifer Meyering, RN, BSN, MS, CCRN

Acquisitions Editor
Bill Lamsback

Product Director
David Moreau

Product Managers
Rosanne Hallowell and Jennifer K. Forestieri

Editorial Assistants
Karen J. Kirk, Jeri O'Shea, Linda K. Ruhf

Art Director
Elaine Kasmer

Illustrator
Bot Roda

Vendor Manager
Cynthia Rudy

Manufacturing Manager
Beth J. Welsh

Production Services
SPi Technologies

Printed in the United States.

6COMPIE010810-020810

ISBN-13: 978-1-4511-0820-0
ISBN-10: 1-4511-0820-6

Contents

Preface   *v*

Joy's NCLEX adventure   *vii*

Part I   Surviving the NCLEX®

1   Preparing for the NCLEX®   3
2   Passing the NCLEX®   21

Part II   Comprehensive tests

3   Comprehensive test 1   33
4   Comprehensive test 2   52
5   Comprehensive test 3   70
6   Comprehensive test 4   89
7   Comprehensive test 5   109
8   Comprehensive test 6   128

Preface

Research shows that the more you become accustomed to the styles and types of questions that may be asked, the more successful you will be on the actual exam. *NCLEX-RN Made Incredibly Easy: 6 Comprehensive Tests* presents 6 NCLEX tests of 75 questions each. These tests simulate the actual NCLEX exam and help you hone your exam preparation skills.

While the overall approach of this book follows the *Incredibly Easy* series design, the questions are tough, and they follow the NCLEX 2010 test plan. The easy-to-use format features questions on the left and answers on the right of the same page. Clear, detailed rationales for both correct and incorrect answers are provided, and each answer provides information on the client needs category, the cognitive level of the question, and the nursing process. In addition, the encouraging words and graphics keep you focused and help build your confidence.

In addition to your nursing knowledge, your test-taking skills can help you pass the exam. This book introduces you to the NCLEX-RN exam structure and covers techniques that will help you learn how to read test questions and understand what they are really asking—skills that are vital to NCLEX success. You also have access to study strategies, such as scheduling study time, maintaining your concentration, and finding the right study space. These all help demystify the process of preparing for, taking, and understanding the results of the NCLEX.

Be proud of your accomplishments and of your decision to prepare yourself well for the NCLEX-RN. You've worked hard to come this far. Now it's time to prepare, to practice, and to succeed!

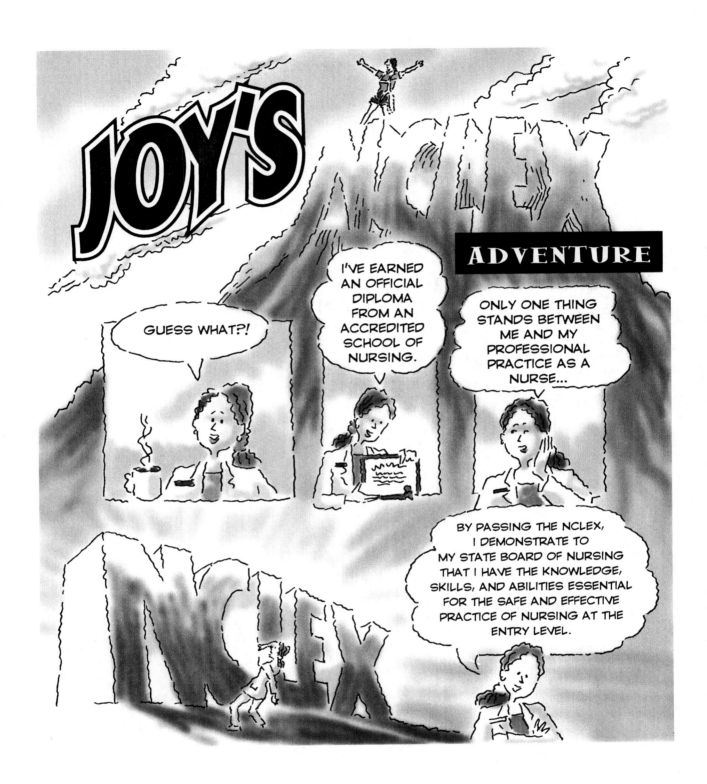

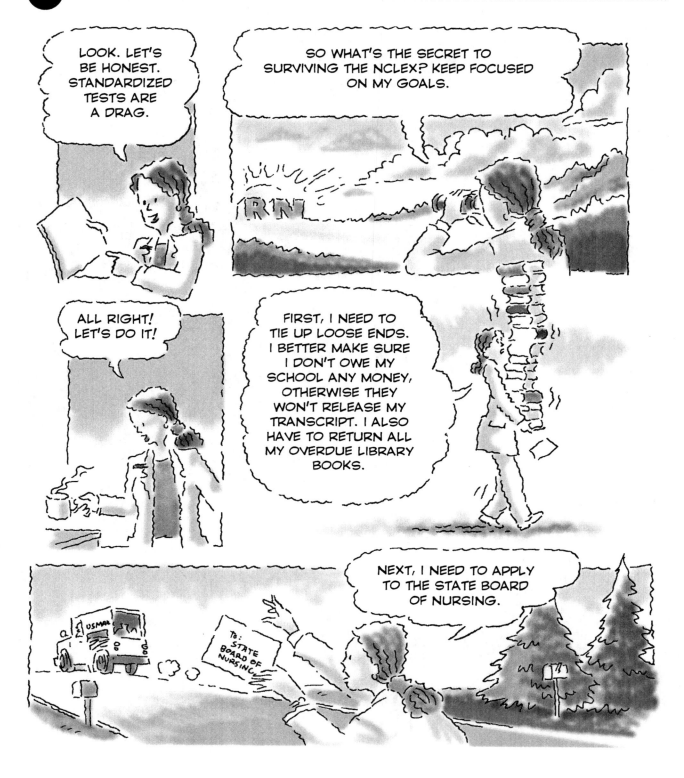

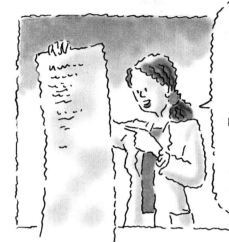

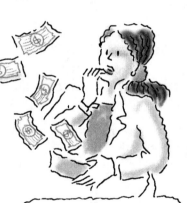

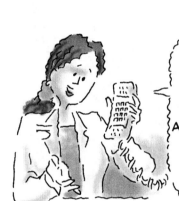

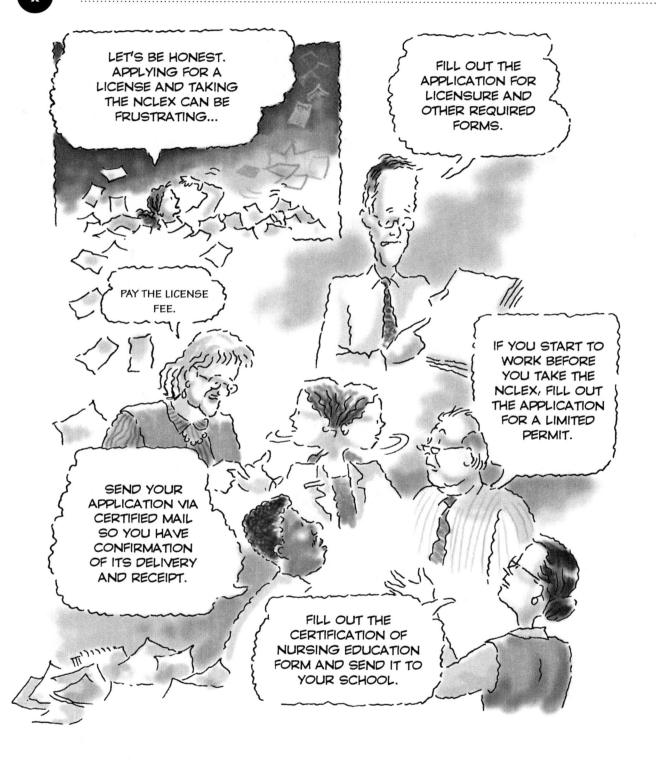

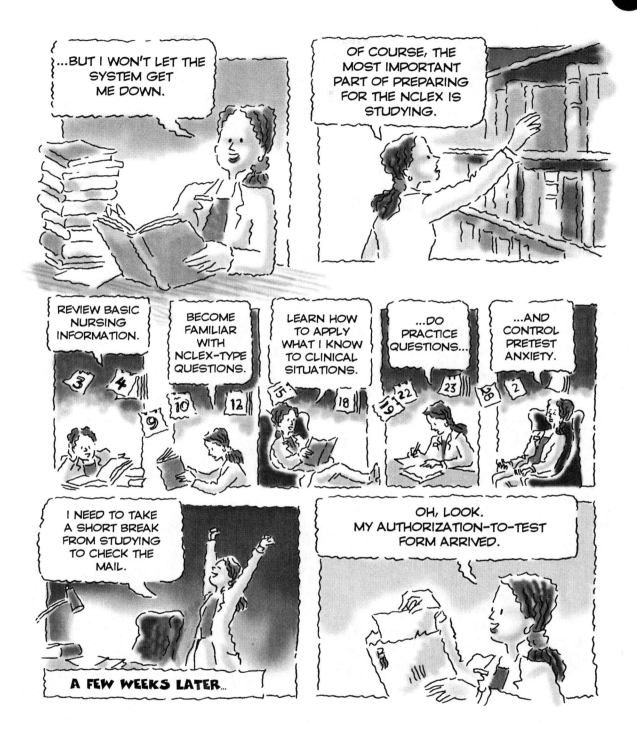

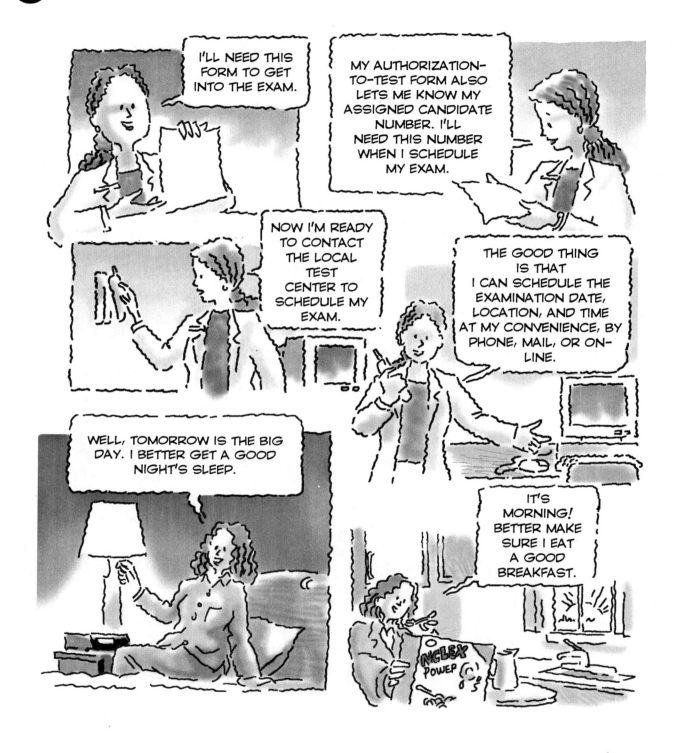

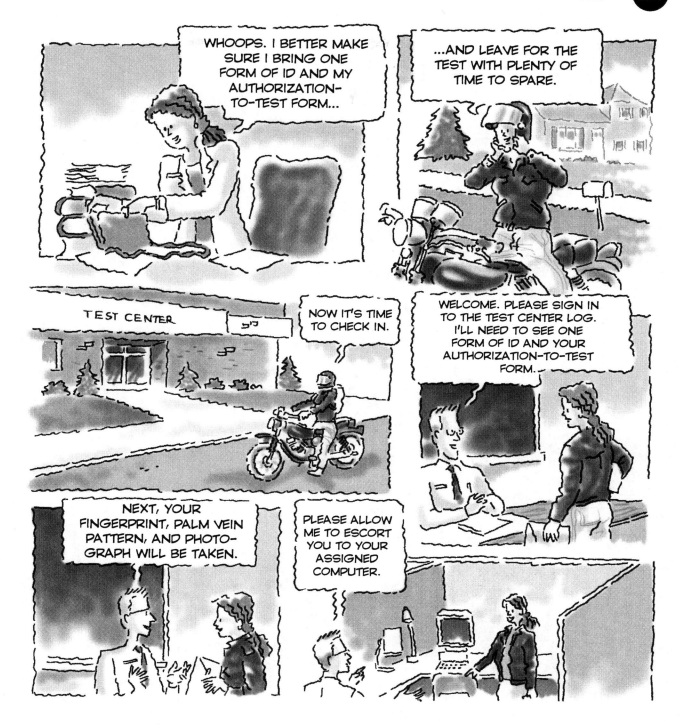

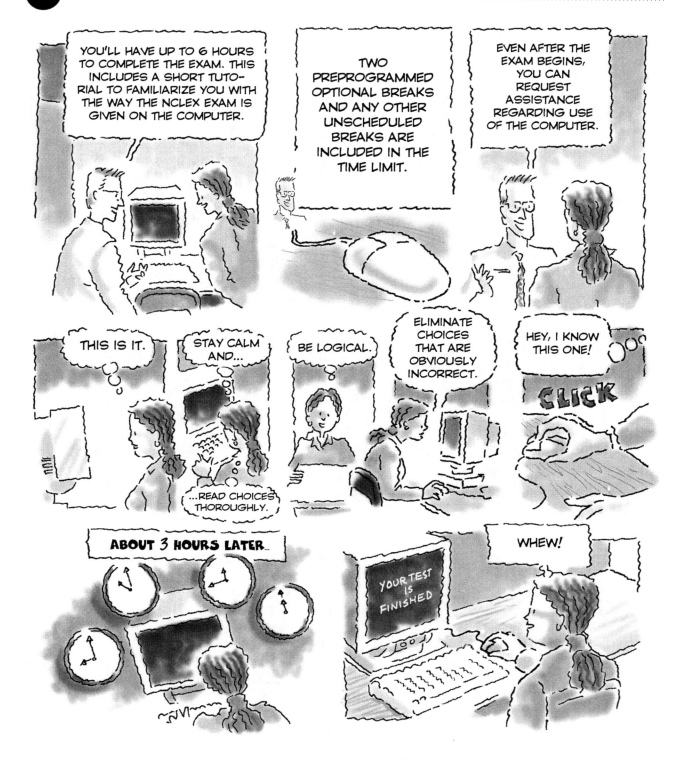

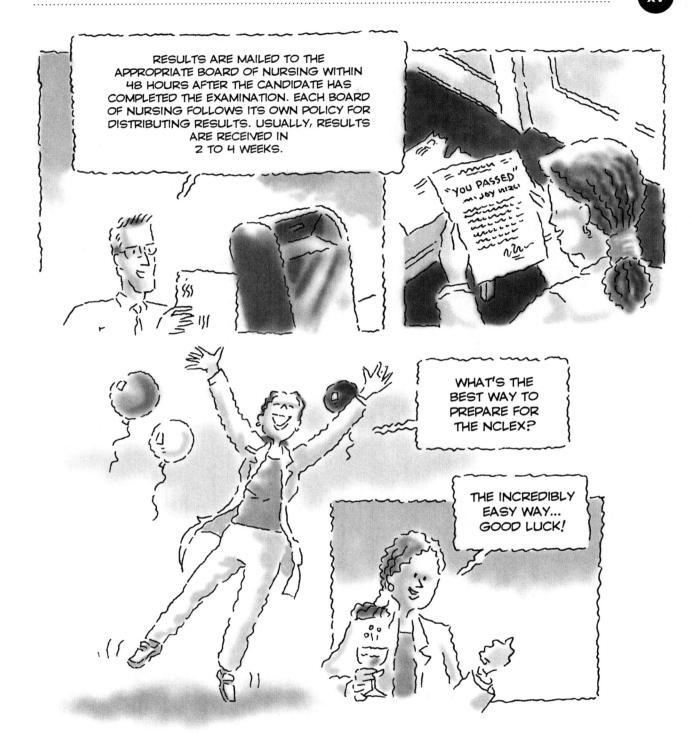

Part I   Surviving the NCLEX®

1   **Preparing for the NCLEX®**   3

2   **Passing the NCLEX®**   21

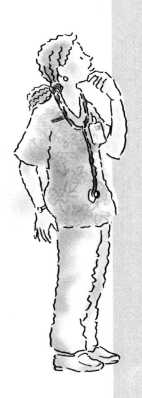

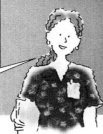

Understanding the NCLEX goals and structure is an important first step in proper preparation for the test. This chapter explains how best to prepare for this important examination.

Chapter 1
Preparing for the NCLEX®

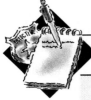

▶ Just the facts

In this chapter, you'll learn:

♦ about the NCLEX and why you must take it

♦ what you need to know about taking the NCLEX by computer

♦ strategies to use when answering NCLEX questions

♦ how to recognize and answer alternate-format questions

♦ how to avoid common mistakes when taking the NCLEX.

NCLEX basics

Passing the National Council Licensure Examination (NCLEX) is an important landmark in your career as a nurse. The first step on your way to passing the NCLEX is to understand what it is and how it's administered.

NCLEX structure

The NCLEX is a test written by nurses who, like most of your nursing instructors, have an advanced degree and clinical expertise in a particular area. Only one small difference distinguishes nurses who write NCLEX questions: They're trained to write questions in a style particular to the NCLEX.

If you've completed an accredited nursing program, you've already taken numerous tests written by nurses with backgrounds and experiences similar to those of the nurses who write for the NCLEX. The test-taking experience you've already gained will help you pass the NCLEX. So your NCLEX review should be just that—a review.

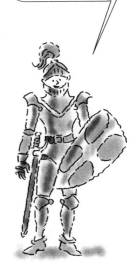

All your experience with testing means you're ready to do battle with this exam!

What's the point of it all?

The NCLEX is designed for one purpose: to determine whether it's appropriate for you to receive a license to practice as a nurse. By passing the NCLEX, you demonstrate that you possess the minimum level of knowledge necessary to practice nursing safely.

Studying abroad

If you completed your nursing education in a foreign country, you must follow certain guidelines to be eligible to work as a registered nurse in the United States. (See *Guidelines for international nurses.*)

Mix 'em up

In nursing school, you probably took courses that were separated into such subjects as pharmacology; nursing leadership; health assessment; adult health; and pediatric, maternal-neonatal, and psychiatric nursing. In contrast, the NCLEX is integrated, meaning that different subjects are mixed together.

As you answer NCLEX questions, you may encounter patients in any stage of life, from neonatal to geriatric. These patients—clients, in NCLEX terminology—may be of any background, and may be completely well or extremely ill, and may have any of a variety of disorders.

Client needs, front and center

The NCLEX draws questions from four categories of client needs that were developed by the *National Council of State Boards of Nursing* (NCSBN), the organization that sponsors and manages the NCLEX. *Client needs categories* ensure that a wide variety of topics appears on every NCLEX examination.

The NCSBN developed client needs categories after conducting a practice analysis of new nurses. All aspects of nursing care observed in the study were broken down into four main categories, some of which were broken down further into subcategories. (See *Client needs categories,* page 6.)

What's the plan?

The categories and subcategories are used to develop the *NCLEX test plan*, the content guidelines for the distribution of test questions. Question writers and the people who put the NCLEX together use the test plan and client needs categories to make sure that a full spectrum of nursing activities is covered in the NCLEX. Client needs categories appear in most NCLEX review and question-and-answer books, including this one. As a test-taker you don't have to concern yourself with client needs categories. You'll see those categories for each question and answer in this book, but they'll be invisible on the actual NCLEX.

Guidelines for international nurses

In order to become eligible to work as a registered nurse (RN) in the United States, you will need to complete several steps. In addition to passing the NCLEX-RN, you may need to obtain a certificate and credentials evaluation from the Commission on Graduates of Foreign Nursing Schools (CGFNS®) and acquire a visa. Since requirements differ from state to state, it's important that you first contact the Board of Nursing in the state where you want to practice nursing.

CGFNS Certification Program

Most states require that you obtain CGFNS certification. This certification requires:
• a review and authentication of your credentials, including your nursing education, registration, and licensure
• a passing score on the CGFNS Qualifying Examination of nursing knowledge
• a passing score on an English language proficiency test.

In order to be eligible to take the CGFNS Qualifying Examination, you must complete a minimum number of classroom and clinical practice hours in medical-surgical nursing, maternal-neonatal nursing, pediatric nursing, and psychiatric and mental health nursing from a government-approved nursing school. You must also be registered as a first-level nurse in your country of education, and currently hold a license as an RN in some jurisdiction.

The CGFNS Qualifying Examination is a paper and pencil test that includes 260 multiple-choice questions. It's administered under controlled testing conditions. Because the test is designed to predict your likelihood of successfully passing the NCLEX-RN exam, it's based on the NCLEX-RN test plan.

You may select from three English proficiency examinations, Test of English as a Foreign Language (TOEFL®), Test of English for International Communication (TOEIC®), or International English Language Testing System (IELTS). Each test has different passing scores and the scores are valid for up to 2 years.

CGFNS credentials evaluation service

This evaluation is a comprehensive report that analyzes and compares your education and licensure with U.S. standards. It's prepared by the CGFNS for a state board of nursing, an immigration office, an employer, or a university. It requires that you complete an application, submit appropriate documentation, and pay a fee.

More information about the CGFNS certification program and credentials evaluation service is available at *www.cgfns.org*.

Visa

You can't legally immigrate to work in the United States without an occupational visa (temporary or permanent) from the United States Citizenship and Immigration Services (USCIS). The visa process is separate from the CGFNS certification process, although some of the same steps are involved. Some visas require prior CGFNS certification and a *VisaScreen*™ Certificate from the International Commission on Healthcare Professions. The *VisaScreen* program involves:
• a credentials review of your nursing education and current registration or licensure
• successful completion of either the CGFNS certification program or the NCLEX-RN to provide proof of nursing knowledge
• a passing score on an approved English language proficiency examination.

Once you successfully complete all parts of the *VisaScreen* program, you will receive a certificate to present to the USCIS. The visa-granting process can take up to a year.

You can obtain more detailed information about visa application at *www.uscis.gov*.

Client needs categories

Each question on the NCLEX is assigned a category based on client needs. This chart lists client needs categories and subcategories and the percentages of each type of question that appears on an NCLEX examination.

Category	Subcategories	Percentage of NCLEX questions
Safe, effective care environment	• Management of care • Safety and infection control	16% to 22% 8% to 14%
Health promotion and maintenance		6% to 12%
Psychosocial integrity		6% to 12%
Physiological integrity	• Basic care and comfort • Pharmacological and parenteral therapies • Reduction of risk potential • Physiological adaptation	6% to 12% 13% to 19% 10% to 16% 11% to 17%

Testing by computer

Like many standardized tests today, the NCLEX is administered by computer. That means you won't be filling in empty circles, sharpening pencils, or erasing frantically. It also means that you must become familiar with computer tests, if you aren't already. Fortunately, the skills required to take the NCLEX on a computer are simple enough to allow you to focus on the questions, not the keyboard.

Q&A

When you take the test, depending on the question format, you'll be presented with a question and four or more possible answers, a blank space in which to enter your answer, a figure on which you'll click the mouse to select the correct area of the figure, a series of charts or exhibits to view in order to select the correct response, items you must prioritize by dragging and dropping them in place, an audio recording to listen to in order to select the correct response, or a question and four graphic options.

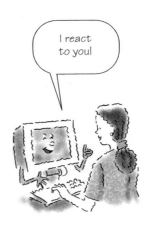

I react to you!

Feeling smart? Think hard!

The NCLEX is a *computer-adaptive test*, meaning that the computer reacts to the answers you give, supplying more difficult questions if you answer correctly, and slightly easier questions if you answer incorrectly. Each test is thus uniquely adapted to the individual test-taker.

A matter of time

You have a great deal of flexibility with the amount of time you spend on individual questions. The examination lasts a maximum of 6 hours, however, so don't waste time. If you fail to answer a set number of questions within 6 hours, the computer will determine that you lack minimum competency.

Most students have plenty of time to complete the test, so take as much time as you need to get the question right without wasting time. Keep moving at a decent pace to help maintain concentration.

Difficult items = Good news

If you find as you progress through the test that the questions seem to be increasingly difficult, it's a good sign. The more questions you answer correctly, the more difficult the questions become.

Some students, though, knowing that questions get progressively harder, focus on the degree of difficulty of subsequent questions to try to figure out if they're answering questions correctly. Avoid the temptation to do this, as this may get you off track.

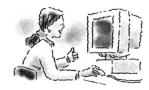

The harder it gets, the better I do.

The finish line

The computer test finishes when one of these events occurs:
• You demonstrate minimum competency, according to the computer program, which calculates with 95% certainty that your ability exceeds the passing standard.
• You demonstrate a lack of minimum competency, according to the computer program.
• You've answered the maximum number of questions (265 total questions).
• You've used the maximum time allowed (6 hours).

Unlocking the NCLEX mystery

In April of 2004, the NCSBN added alternate-format items to the exam. However, most of the questions on the NCLEX are four-option, multiple-choice items with only one correct answer. Certain strategies can help you understand and answer any type of NCLEX question.

Alternate formats

The first type of alternate-format item is the *multiple-response, multiple-choice question.* Unlike a traditional multiple-choice question, each multiple-response, multiple-choice question has more than one correct answer for every question, and it may contain more than four possible answer options. You'll recognize this type of question because it will ask you to select *all* answers that apply—not just the best answer (as may be requested in the more traditional multiple-choice questions).

No points for partials

Keep in mind that for each multiple-response, multiple-choice question, you must select at least one answer and you must select all correct answers for the item to be counted as correct. On the NCLEX, there's no partial credit in the scoring of these items.

Don't go blank!

The second type of alternate-format item is the *fill-in-the-blank*. These questions require you to provide the answer yourself, rather than select it from a list of options. You will perform a calculation, then type your answer (a number without any words, units of measurement, commas, or spaces) in the blank space provided after the question. Rules for rounding are included in the question stem if appropriate. A calculator button is provided so you can easily do your calculations electronically.

Master that mouse!

The third type of alternate-format item is a question that asks you to identify an area on an illustration or graphic. For these so-called *"hotspot"* questions, the computerized exam will ask you to place your cursor and click over the correct area on an illustration. Try to be as precise as possible when marking the location. As with the fill-in-the-blanks, the identification questions on the computerized exam may require extremely precise answers to be considered correct.

Chart smarts

The fourth type of alternate-format item is the *chart/exhibit* format. Here you'll be given a problem, then a series of small screens containing additional information you'll need in order to answer the question. By clicking on the Tab button, you can access each screen in turn. Your answer can then be chosen from four multiple-choice answer options.

All in order

The fifth type of alternate-format item involves prioritizing or placing in correct order a series of statements, using a *drag-and-drop* technique. You'll decide which of the given options is first, click and hold it with the mouse, then drag it into the first box given underneath and drop it into place. You'll repeat this process until you've placed all the available options in the lower boxes.

Now hear this!

The sixth alternate-format item type is the *audio item* format. You'll be given a set of headphones and you'll be asked to listen to an audio clip and select the correct answer from four options. You'll need to select the correct answer on the computer screen as you would with the traditional multiple-choice questions.

Picture perfect

The final alternate-format item type is the *graphic option* question. This varies from the exhibit format type because in the graphic option, your answer choices will be graphics, such as ECG strips. You'll have to select the appropriate graphic to answer the question presented.

The standard's still the standard

The NCSBN hasn't yet established a percentage of alternate-format items to be administered to each candidate. In fact, your exam may contain only one alternate-format item. So relax; the standard, four-option, multiple-choice format questions compose the bulk of the test. (See *Sample NCLEX questions,* pages 10–12.)

Understanding the question

NCLEX questions are usually long. As a result, it's easy to feel overwhelmed with information. To focus on the question, apply proven strategies for answering NCLEX questions, including:
- determining what the question is asking
- determining relevant facts about the client
- rephrasing the question in your mind
- choosing the best option(s) before entering your answer.

Determine what the question is asking

Read the question twice. If the answer isn't apparent, rephrase the question in simpler, more personal terms. Breaking down the question into easier, less intimidating terms may help you to focus more accurately on the correct answer.

Give it a try

For example, a question might be, "A 74-year-old client with a history of heart failure is admitted to the coronary care unit with pulmonary edema. He's intubated and placed on a mechanical ventilator. Which parameter should the nurse monitor closely to assess the client's response to a bolus dose of furosemide (Lasix) I.V.?"

The options for this question—numbered from 1 to 4—may be:
1. Daily weight
2. 24-hour intake and output
3. Serum sodium levels
4. Hourly urine output

Sample NCLEX questions

Sometimes, getting used to the test format is as important as knowing the material covered. Try your hand at these sample questions and you'll have a leg up when you take the real test!

Sample four-option, multiple-choice question

A client's arterial blood gas (ABG) results are as follows: pH, 7.16; $Paco_2$, 80 mm Hg; Pao_2, 46 mm Hg; HCO_3^-, 24 mEq/L; Sao_2, 81%. This ABG result represents which condition?

1. Metabolic acidosis
2. Metabolic alkalosis
3. Respiratory acidosis
4. Respiratory alkalosis

Correct answer: 3

Sample multiple-response, multiple-choice question

The nurse is caring for a 45-year-old married client who has undergone hemicolectomy for colon cancer. The client has two children. Which concepts about families should the nurse keep in mind when providing care for this client? Select all that apply:

1. Illness in one family member can affect all members.
2. Family roles don't change because of illness.
3. A family member may have more than one role in the family.
4. Children typically aren't affected by adult illness.
5. The effects of an illness on a family depend on the stage of the family's life cycle.
6. Changes in sleeping and eating patterns may be signs of stress in a family.

Correct answer: 1, 3, 5, 6

Sample fill-in-the-blank calculation question

An infant who weighs 8 kg is to receive ampicillin 25 mg/kg I.V. every 6 hours. How many milligrams should the nurse administer per dose? Record your answer using a whole number.

_____ milligrams

Correct answer: 200

Sample hotspot question

A client has a history of aortic stenosis. Identify the area where the nurse should place the stethoscope to best hear the murmur.

Correct answer:

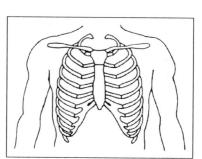

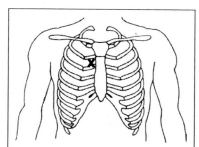

Sample NCLEX questions (continued)

Sample chart/exhibit question

A 3-year-old client is being treated for severe status asthmaticus. After reviewing the progress notes (shown below), the nurse should determine that this client is being treated for which condition?

Progress notes	
4/5/10	Pt. was acutely restless, diaphoretic, and with
0600	dyspnea at 0530. Dr. T. Smith notified and
	ordered ABG analysis. ABG drawn from (R)
	radial artery. Stat results as follows: pH 7.28,
	$Paco_2$ 55 mm Hg, HCO_3- 26 mEg/L. Dr. Smith
	with pt. now. —————— J. Collins, R.N.

1. Metabolic acidosis
2. Respiratory alkalosis
3. Respiratory acidosis
4. Metabolic alkalosis

Correct answer: 3

Sample drag-and-drop question

When teaching an antepartal client about the passage of the fetus through the birth canal during labor, the nurse describes the cardinal mechanisms of labor. Place these events in the sequence in which they occur. Use all the options.

1. Flexion
2. External rotation
3. Descent
4. Expulsion
5. Internal rotation
6. Extension

Correct answer:

3. Descent
1. Flexion
5. Internal rotation
6. Extension
2. External rotation
4. Expulsion

Sample NCLEX questions *(continued)*

Sample audio item question

Listen to the audio clip. What sound do you hear in the bases of this client with heart failure?

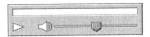

1. Crackles
2. Rhonchi
3. Wheezes
4. Pleural friction rub

Correct answer: 1

Sample graphic option question

Which electrocardiogram strip should the nurse document as sinus tachycardia?

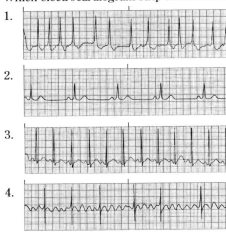

1.

2.

3.

4.

Correct answer: 3

Hocus, focus on the question

Read the question again, ignoring all details except what's being asked. Focus on the last line of the question. It asks you to select the appropriate assessment for monitoring a client who received a bolus of furosemide I.V.

Determine what facts about the client are relevant

Next, sort out the relevant client information. Start by asking whether any of the information provided about the client isn't relevant. For instance, do you need to know that the client has been admitted to the coronary care unit? Probably not; his reaction to I.V. furosemide won't be affected by his location in the hospital.

Determine what you do know about the client. In the example, you know that:

• he just received an I.V. bolus of furosemide, a crucial fact
• he has pulmonary edema, the most fundamental aspect of the client's underlying condition
• he's intubated and placed on a mechanical ventilator, suggesting that his pulmonary edema is serious
• he's 74 years old and has a history of heart failure, a fact that may or may not be relevant.

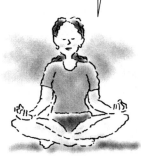

Focusing on what the question is really asking can help you choose the correct answer.

Rephrase the question

After you've determined relevant information about the client and the question being asked, consider rephrasing the question to make it more clear. Eliminate jargon and put the question in simpler, more personal terms. Here's how you might rephrase the question in the example: "My client has pulmonary edema. He requires intubation and mechanical ventilation. He's 74 years old and has a history of heart failure. He received an I.V. bolus of furosemide. What assessment parameter should I monitor?"

Choose the best option

Armed with all the information you now have, it's time to select an option. You know that the client received an I.V. bolus of furosemide, a diuretic. You know that monitoring fluid intake and output is a key nursing intervention for a client taking a diuretic, a fact that eliminates options 1 and 3 (daily weight and serum sodium levels), narrowing the answer down to option 2 or 4 (24-hour intake and output or hourly urine output).

Can I use a lifeline?

You also know that the drug was administered by I.V. bolus, suggesting a rapid effect. (In fact, furosemide administered by I.V. bolus takes effect almost immediately.) Monitoring the client's 24-hour intake and output would be appropriate for assessing the effects of repeated doses of furosemide. Hourly urine output, however, is most appropriate in this situation because it monitors the immediate effect of this rapid-acting drug.

Key strategies

Regardless of the type of question, four key strategies will help you determine the correct answer for each question. These strategies are:

 considering the nursing process

referring to Maslow's hierarchy of needs

reviewing patient safety

reflecting on principles of therapeutic communication.

Nursing process

One of the ways to answer a question is to apply the nursing process. Steps in the nursing process include:
- assessment
- diagnosis
- planning
- implementation
- evaluation.

Process pointers

The nursing process may provide insights that help you analyze a question. According to the nursing process, assessment comes before analysis, which comes before planning, which comes before implementation, which comes before evaluation.

You're halfway to the correct answer when you encounter a four-option, multiple-choice question that asks you to assess the situation and then provides two assessment options and two implementation options. You can immediately eliminate the implementation options, which then gives you, at worst, a 50-50 chance of selecting the correct answer. Use the following sample question to apply the nursing process:

A client returns from an endoscopic procedure during which he was sedated. Before offering the client food, which action should the nurse take?
1. Assess the client's respiratory status.
2. Check the client's gag reflex.
3. Place the client in a side-lying position.
4. Have the client drink a few sips of water.

Assess before intervening

According to the nursing process, the nurse must assess a client before performing an intervention. Does the question indicate

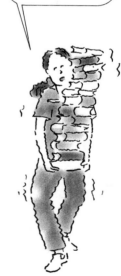

Say it 1,000 times: Studying for the NCLEX is fun... studying for the NCLEX is fun...

that the client has been properly assessed? No, it doesn't. Therefore, you can eliminate options 3 and 4 because they're both interventions.

That leaves options 1 and 2, both of which are assessments. Your nursing knowledge should tell you the correct answer—in this case, option 2. The sedation required for an endoscopic procedure may impair the client's gag reflex, so you would assess the gag reflex before giving food to the client to reduce the risk of aspiration and airway obstruction.

Watch phrasing

Why not select option 1, assessing the client's respiratory status? You might select this option but the question is specifically asking about offering the client food, an action that wouldn't be taken if the client's respiratory status was at all compromised. In this case, you're making a judgment based on the phrase, "Before offering the client food." If the question was trying to test your knowledge of respiratory depression following an endoscopic procedure, it probably wouldn't mention a function—such as giving food to a client—that clearly occurs only after the client's respiratory status has been stabilized.

Maslow's hierarchy

Knowledge of Maslow's hierarchy of needs can be a vital tool for establishing priorities on the NCLEX. Maslow's theory states that physiologic needs are the most basic human needs of all. Only after physiologic needs have been met can safety concerns be addressed. Only after safety concerns are met can concerns involving love and belonging be addressed, and so forth. Apply the principles of Maslow's hierarchy of needs to the following sample question:

A client complains of severe pain 2 days after surgery. Which action should the nurse perform first?
1. Offer reassurance to the client that he will feel less pain tomorrow.
2. Allow the client time to verbalize his feelings.
3. Check the client's vital signs.
4. Administer an analgesic.

Phys before psych

In this example, two of the options—3 and 4—address physiologic needs. Options 1 and 2 address psychosocial concerns. According to Maslow, physiologic needs must be met before psychosocial needs, so you can eliminate options 1 and 2.

Final elimination

Now, use your nursing knowledge to choose the best answer from the two remaining options. In this case, option 3 is correct because the client's vital signs should be checked before administering an analgesic (assessment before intervention). When prioritizing according to Maslow's hierarchy, remember your ABCs—airway, breathing, circulation—to help you further prioritize. Check for a patent airway before addressing breathing. Check breathing before checking the health of the cardiovascular system.

Tricky, tricky

Just because an option appears on the NCLEX doesn't mean it's a viable choice for the client referred to in the question. Always examine your choice in light of your knowledge and experience. Ask yourself, "Does this choice make sense for this client?" Allow yourself to eliminate choices—even ones that might normally take priority—if they don't make sense for a particular client's situation.

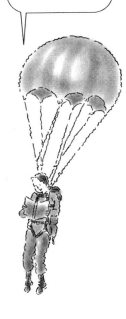

Patient safety takes high priority on the NCLEX.

Patient safety

As you might expect, patient safety takes high priority on the NCLEX. You'll encounter many questions that can be answered by asking yourself, "Which answer will best ensure the safety of this client?" Use patient safety criteria for situations involving laboratory values, drug administration, activities of daily living, or nursing care procedures.

Client first, equipment second

You may encounter a question in which some options address the client and others address the equipment. When in doubt, select an option relating to the client; never place equipment before a client.

For instance, suppose a question asks what the nurse should do first when entering a client's room where an infusion pump alarm is sounding. If two options deal with the infusion pump, one with the infusion tubing, and another with the client's catheter insertion site, select the one relating to the client's catheter insertion site. Always check the client first; the equipment can wait.

Therapeutic communication

Some NCLEX questions focus on the nurse's ability to communicate effectively with the client. Therapeutic communication incorporates verbal or nonverbal responses and involves:

- listening to the client
- understanding the client's needs
- promoting clarification and insight about the client's condition.

Room for improvement

Like other NCLEX questions, those dealing with therapeutic communication require choosing the best response. First, eliminate options that indicate the use of poor therapeutic communication techniques, such as those in which the nurse:
- tells the client what to do without regard to the client's feelings or desires (the "do this" response)
- asks a question that can be answered "yes" or "no," or with another one-syllable response
- seeks reasons for the client's behavior
- implies disapproval of the client's behavior
- offers false reassurances
- attempts to interpret the client's behavior rather than allowing the client to verbalize his own feelings
- offers a response that focuses on the nurse, not the client.

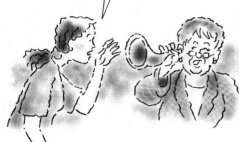

I said that some exam questions will focus on good therapeutic COMMUNICATION!

Ah, that's better!

When answering NCLEX questions, look for responses that:
- allow the client time to think and reflect
- encourage the client to talk
- encourage the client to describe a particular experience
- reflect that the nurse has listened to the client, such as through paraphrasing the client's response.

Avoiding pitfalls

Even the most knowledgeable students can get tripped up on certain NCLEX questions. (See *A tricky question*.) Students commonly cite three areas that can be difficult for unwary test-takers:

 knowing the difference between the NCLEX and the "real world"

 delegating care

 knowing laboratory values.

NCLEX versus the real world

Some students who take the NCLEX have extensive practical experience in health care. For example, many test-takers have

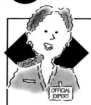

> ### *Advice from the experts*
>
> ## A tricky question
>
> The NCLEX occasionally asks a particular kind of question called the "further teaching" question, which involves patient-teaching situations. These questions can be tricky. You'll have to choose the response that suggests that the patient has *not* learned the correct information. Here's an example:
>
> **37.** A client undergoes a total hip replacement. Which statement by the client indicates that he requires further teaching?
>
> 1. "I'll need to keep several pillows between my legs at night."
> 2. "I'll need to remember not to cross my legs. It's such a bad habit."
> 3. "The occupational therapist is showing me how to use a 'sock puller' to help me get dressed."
> 4. "I don't know if I'll be able to get off that low toilet seat at home by myself."
>
> The answer you should choose here is option 4 because it indicates that the client has a poor understanding of the precautions required after a total hip replacement and that he needs further teaching. *Remember:* If you see the phrase *further teaching* or *further instruction*, you're looking for a wrong answer by the patient.

worked as licensed practical nurses or nursing assistants. In one of those capacities, test-takers might have been exposed to less than optimum clinical practice and may carry those experiences over to the NCLEX.

However, the NCLEX is a textbook examination—not a test of clinical skills. Take the NCLEX with the understanding that what happens in the real world may differ from what the NCLEX and your nursing school say should happen.

Don't take shortcuts

If you've had practical experience in health care, you may know a quicker way to perform a procedure or tricks to get by when you don't have the right equipment. Situations such as staff shortages may force you to improvise. On the NCLEX, such scenarios can lead to trouble. Always check your practical experiences against textbook nursing care, taking care to select the response that follows the textbook.

> Remember, this is the real world. The NCLEX may not always reflect what happens in it.

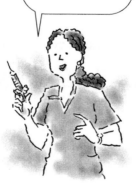

Delegating care

On the NCLEX, you may encounter questions that assess your ability to delegate care. Delegating care involves coordinating

the efforts of other health care workers to provide effective care for your client. On the NCLEX, you may be asked to assign duties to:
• licensed practical nurses or licensed vocational nurses
• direct care workers, such as nursing assistants and personal care aides
• other support staff, such as nutrition assistants and house-keepers.

In addition, you'll be asked to decide when to notify a physician, a social worker, or another hospital staff member. In each case, you'll have to decide when, where, and how to delegate.

Shoulds and shouldn'ts

As a general rule, it's okay to delegate actions that involve stable clients or standard, unchanging procedures. Bathing, feeding, dressing, and transferring clients are examples of procedures that can be delegated.

Be careful not to delegate complicated or complex activities. In addition, don't delegate activities that involve assessment, evaluation, or your own nursing judgment. On the NCLEX and in the real world, these duties fall squarely on your shoulders. Make sure that you take primary responsibility for assessing and evaluating the client and for making decisions about the client's care. Never hand off those responsibilities to someone with less training.

Calling in reinforcements

Deciding when to notify a physician, a social worker, or another hospital staff member is an important element of nursing care. On the NCLEX, however, choices that involve notifying the physician are usually incorrect. Remember that the NCLEX wants to see you, the nurse, at work.

If you're sure the correct answer is to notify the physician, though, make sure the client's safety has been addressed before notifying a physician or another staff member. On the NCLEX, the client's safety has a higher priority than notifying other health care providers.

Knowing laboratory values

Some NCLEX questions supply laboratory results without indicating normal levels. As a result, answering questions involving laboratory values requires you to have the normal range of the most common laboratory values memorized to make an informed decision. (See *Normal laboratory values.*)

> ## Normal laboratory values
>
> • Blood urea nitrogen: 8 to 25 mg/dl
> • Creatinine: 0.6 to 1.5 mg/dl
> • Sodium: 135 to 145 mmol/L
> • Potassium: 3.5 to 5.5 mEq/L
> • Chloride: 97 to 110 mmol/L
> • Glucose (fasting plasma): 70 to 110 mg/dl
> • Hemoglobin
>   Male: 13.8 to 17.2 g/dl
>   Female: 12.1 to 15.1 g/dl
> • Hematocrit
>   Male: 40.7% to 50.3%
>   Female: 36.1% to 44.3%

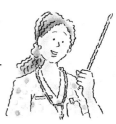

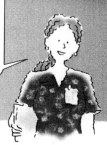

As you count down the weeks, days, and finally hours to the NCLEX, refer back to the information in this chapter. It's a recipe for NCLEX success!

Chapter 2
Passing the NCLEX®

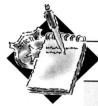

Just the facts

In this chapter, you'll learn:

◆ In this chapter, you'll learn:

◆ how to properly prepare for the NCLEX

◆ how to concentrate during difficult study times

◆ ways to make more effective use of your time

◆ why creative studying strategies can enhance learning

◆ how to get the most out of NCLEX practice tests.

Most students pass the NCLEX on the first try. I know you can, too!

Study preparations

If you're like most people preparing to take the test, you're probably feeling nervous, anxious, or concerned. Keep in mind that most test-takers pass the NCLEX the first time around.

Passing the test won't happen by accident, though; you'll need to prepare carefully and efficiently. To help jump-start your preparations:
• determine your strengths and weaknesses
• create a study schedule
• set realistic goals
• find an effective study space
• think positively
• start studying sooner rather than later.

Strengths and weaknesses

Most students recognize that, even at the end of their nursing studies, they know more about some topics than others. Because the NCLEX covers a broad range of material, you should make some decisions about how intensively you'll review each topic.

Make a list

Base those decisions on a list. Divide a sheet of paper in half vertically. On one side, list topics you think you know well. On the other side, list topics you need to review. Pay no attention if one side is longer than the other. When you're done studying, you'll feel strong in every area.

Where the list comes from

To make sure your list reflects a comprehensive view of all the areas you studied in school, look at the contents page in the front of this book. For each topic listed, place it in the "know well" column or "needs review" column. Separating content areas this way shows immediately which topics need less study time and which need more time.

Scheduling study time

Study when you're most alert. Most people can identify a period of the day when they feel most alert. If you feel most alert and energized in the morning, for example, set aside sections of time in the morning for topics that need a lot of review. Then you can use the evening, a time of lesser alertness, for topics that need some refreshing. The opposite is true as well; if you're more alert in the evening, study difficult topics at that time.

I'll cover difficult topics in the morning when I'm more alert.

What and when

Set up a basic schedule for studying. Using a calendar or organizer, determine how much time remains before you'll take the NCLEX. (See *2 to 3 months before the NCLEX*.) Fill in the remaining days with specific times and topics to be studied. For example, you might schedule the respiratory system on a Tuesday morning and the GI system that afternoon. Remember to schedule difficult topics during your most alert times.

Keep in mind that you shouldn't fill each day with studying. Be realistic and set aside time for normal activities. Try to create ample study time before the NCLEX and then stick to the schedule. Allow some extra time in the schedule in case you get behind or come across a topic that requires extra review.

Keep goals manageable

Part of creating a schedule means setting goals you can accomplish. You no doubt studied a great deal in nursing school, and by now you have a sense of your own capabilities. Ask yourself, "How much can I cover in a day?" Set that amount of time aside and then stay on task. You'll feel better about yourself—and your

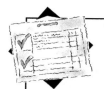

To-do list

2 to 3 months before the NCLEX

With 2 to 3 months remaining before you plan to take the examination, take these steps:
• Establish a study schedule. Set aside ample time to study but also leave time for social activities, exercise, family or personal responsibilities, and other matters.
• Become knowledgeable about the NCLEX-RN examination, its content, the types of questions it asks, and the testing format.
• Begin studying your notes, texts, and other study materials.
• Take some NCLEX practice questions to help you diagnose strengths and weaknesses as well as to become familiar with NCLEX-style questions.

chances of passing the NCLEX—when you meet your goals regularly.

Study space

Find a space conducive to effective learning and then study there. Whatever you do, don't study with a television on in the room. Instead, find a quiet, inviting study space that:
• is located in a quiet, convenient place, away from normal traffic patterns
• contains a solid chair that encourages good posture (Avoid studying in bed; you'll be more likely to fall asleep and not accomplish your goals.)
• uses comfortable, soft lighting with which you can see clearly without eye strain
• has a temperature between 65° and 70° F
• contains flowers or green plants, familiar photos or paintings, and easy access to soft, instrumental background music.

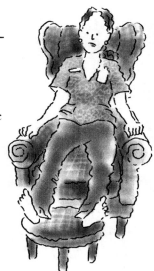

This chair invites slacking, not studying! You should find a chair that encourages good posture instead.

Accentuate the positive

Consider taping positive messages around your study space. Make signs with words of encouragement, such as, "You can do it!" "Keep studying!" and "Remember the goal!" These upbeat messages can help keep you going when your attention begins to waver.

Maintaining concentration

When you're faced with reviewing the amount of information covered by the NCLEX, it's easy to become distracted and lose your concentration. When you lose concentration, you make less effective use of valuable study time. To help stay focused, keep these tips in mind:

• Alternate the order of the subjects you study during the day to add variety to your study. Try alternating between topics you find most interesting and those you find least interesting.

• Approach your studying with enthusiasm, sincerity, and determination.

• Once you've decided to study, begin immediately. Don't let anything interfere with your thought processes once you've begun.

• Concentrate on accomplishing one task at a time, to the exclusion of everything else.

• Don't try to do two things at once, such as studying and watching television or conversing with friends.

• Work continuously without interruption for a while, but don't study for such a long period that the whole experience becomes grueling or boring.

• Allow time for periodic breaks to give yourself a change of pace. Use these breaks to ease your transition into studying a new topic.

• When studying in the evening, wind down from your studies slowly. Don't progress directly from studying to sleeping.

Taking care of yourself

Never neglect your physical and mental well-being in favor of longer study hours. Maintaining physical and mental health is critical for success in taking the NCLEX. (See *4 to 6 weeks before the NCLEX.*)

A few simple rules

You can increase your likelihood of passing the test by following these simple health rules:

• Get plenty of rest. You can't think deeply or concentrate for long periods when you're tired.

• Drink enough noncaffeinated beverages. Mild dehydration increases the effort required to concentrate and reason while distracting attention through feelings of fatigue and thirst.

• Eat nutritious meals. Maintaining your energy level is impossible when you're undernourished.

To-do list

4 to 6 weeks before the NCLEX

With 4 to 6 weeks remaining before you plan to take the examination, take these steps:

• Focus on your areas of weakness. That way, you'll have time to review these areas again before the test date.

• Find a study partner or form a study group.

• Take a practice test to gauge your skill level early.

• Take time to eat, sleep, exercise, and socialize to avoid burnout.

• Exercise regularly. Regular exercise, preferably 30 minutes daily, helps you work harder and think more clearly. As a result, you'll study more efficiently and increase the likelihood of success.

Memory powers, activate!

If you're having trouble concentrating but would rather push through than take a break, try making your studying more active by reading out loud. Active studying can renew your powers of concentration. By reading review material out loud to yourself, you're engaging your ears as well as your eyes—and making your studying a more active process. Hearing the material out loud also fosters memory and subsequent recall.

You can also rewrite in your own words a few of the more difficult concepts you're reviewing. Explaining these concepts in writing forces you to think through the material and can jump-start your memory.

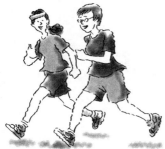

A short jog now will help us concentrate later.

Study schedule

When you were creating your schedule, you might have asked yourself, "How long should I study? One hour at a stretch? Two hours? Three?" To make the best use of your study time, you'll need to answer those questions.

Optimum study time

Consider studying in 20- to 30-minute intervals with a short break in-between. You remember the material you study at the beginning and end of a session best and tend to remember less material studied in the middle of the session. The total length of time in each study session depends on you and the amount of material you need to cover.

To thine own self be true

So what's the answer? It doesn't matter as long as you determine what's best for *you*. At the beginning of your NCLEX study schedule, try study periods of varying lengths. Pay close attention to those that seem more successful.

Remember that you're a trained nurse who is competent at assessment. Think of yourself as a patient, and assess your own progress. Then implement the strategy that works best for you.

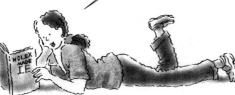

I've found that hour-and-a-half sessions work best for me.

Finding time to study

So does that mean that short sections of time are useless? Not at all. We all have spaces in our day that might otherwise be dead time. (See *1 week before the NCLEX*.) These are perfect times to review for the NCLEX but not to cover new material because by the time you get deep into new material, your time will be over. Always keep some flashcards or a small notebook handy for situations when you have a few extra minutes.

You'll be amazed how many short sessions you can find in a day and how much reviewing you can do in 5 minutes. The following places offer short stretches of time you can use:
• eating breakfast
• waiting for, or riding on, a train or bus
• waiting in line at the bank, post office, bookstore, or other places
• using exercise equipment, such as a treadmill.

Creative studying

Even when you study in a perfect study space and concentrate better than ever, studying for the NCLEX can get a little, well, dull. Even people with terrific study habits occasionally feel bored or sluggish. That is why it's important to have some creative tricks in your study bag to liven up your studying during those down times.

Creative studying doesn't have to be hard work. It involves making efforts to alter your study habits a bit. Some techniques that might help include studying with a partner or group and creating flash cards or other audiovisual study tools.

Study partners

Studying with a partner or group of students (3 or 4 students at most) can be an excellent way to energize your studying. Working with a partner allows you to test each other on the material you've reviewed. Your partner can give you encouragement and motivation. Perhaps most important, working with a partner can provide a welcome break from solitary studying.

Be choosy

Exercise some care when choosing a study partner or assembling a study group. A partner who doesn't fit

To-do list

1 week before the NCLEX

With 1 week remaining before the NCLEX examination, take these steps:
• Take a review test to measure your progress.
• Record key ideas and principles on note cards or audiotapes.
• Rest, eat well, and avoid thinking about the examination during nonstudy times.
• Treat yourself to one special event. You've been working hard, and you deserve it!

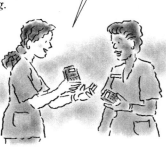

Find a partner with similar goals and strengths. But remember to stay focused!

your needs won't help you make the most of your study time. Look for a partner who:

• possesses similar goals to yours. For example, someone taking the NCLEX at approximately the same date who feels the same sense of urgency as you do might make an excellent partner.

• possesses about the same level of knowledge as you. Tutoring someone can sometimes help you learn, but partnering should be give-and-take so both partners can gain knowledge.

• can study without excess chatting or interruptions. Socializing is an important part of creative study, but remember, you've still got to pass the NCLEX—so stay serious!

Audiovisual tools

Flash cards and other audiovisual tools foster retention and make learning and reviewing fun.

Flash Gordon? No, it's Flash Card!

Flash cards can provide you with an excellent study tool. The process of writing material on a flash card will help you remember it. In addition, flash cards are small and easily portable, perfect for those 5-minute slivers of time that show up during the day.

Creating a flash card should be fun. Use magic markers, highlighters, and other colorful tools to make them visually stimulating. The more effort you put into creating your flash cards, the better you'll remember the material contained on the cards.

Other visual tools

Flowcharts, drawings, diagrams, and other image-oriented study aids can also help you learn material more effectively. Substituting images for text can be a great way to give your eyes a break and recharge your brain. Remember to use vivid colors to make your creations visually engaging.

Hear's the thing

If you learn more effectively when you hear information rather than see it, consider recording key ideas using a handheld tape recorder. Recording information helps promote memory because you say the information aloud when taping and then listen to it when playing it back. Like flash cards, tapes are portable and perfect for those short study periods during the day. (See *The day before the NCLEX*.)

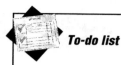

To-do list

The day before the NCLEX

With 1 day before the NCLEX examination, take these steps:

• Drive to the test site, review traffic patterns, and find out where to park. If your route to the test site occurs during heavy traffic or if you're expecting bad weather, set aside extra time to ensure prompt arrival.

• Do something relaxing during the day.

• Avoid concentrating on the test.

• Eat and drink well and avoid dwelling on the NCLEX during nonstudy periods.

• Call a supportive friend or relative for some last-minute words of encouragement.

• Get plenty of rest the night before and allow for plenty of time in the morning.

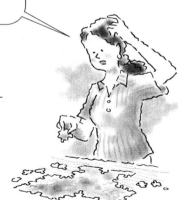

Charts, drawings, and diagrams make concepts less puzzling.

Practice tests

Practice questions should constitute an important part of your NCLEX study strategy. Practice questions can improve your studying by helping you review material and familiarizing yourself with the exact style of questions you'll encounter on the NCLEX.

Practice at the beginning

Consider working through some practice questions as soon as you begin studying for the NCLEX. If you score well, you probably know the material contained in that chapter fairly well and can spend less time reviewing that particular topic. If you have trouble with the questions, spend extra study time on that topic.

You're getting there

Practice questions can also provide an excellent means of marking your progress. Don't worry if you have trouble answering the first few practice questions you take; you'll need time to adjust to the way the questions are asked. Eventually you'll become accustomed to the question format and begin to focus more on the questions themselves.

If you make practice questions a regular part of your study regimen, you'll be able to notice areas in which you're improving. You can then adjust your study time accordingly.

Practice makes perfect

As you near the examination date, continue to answer practice questions, but also set aside time to take an entire NCLEX practice test. (We've included six in this book.) That way, you'll know exactly what to expect. (See *The day of the NCLEX*.) The more you know ahead of time, the better you're likely to do on the NCLEX.

Taking an entire practice test is also a way to gauge your progress. When you find yourself answering questions correctly, it will give you the confidence you need to conquer the real NCLEX.

To-do list

The day of the NCLEX

On the day of the NCLEX examination, take these steps:
• Get up early.
• Wear comfortable clothes, preferably with layers you can adjust to fit the room temperature.
• Drink a glass of water and eat a small nutritious breakfast.
• Leave your house early.
• Arrive at the test site early with the required paperwork in hand.
• Avoid looking at your notes as you wait for your computer test.
• Listen carefully to the instructions given before entering the test room.
• Succeed, succeed, *succeed!*

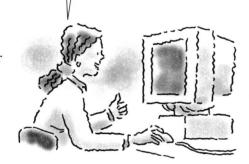

Because I've taken lots of practice tests, I understand how the questions work.

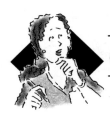

Quick quiz

1. The best time to study is:
   A. in the morning.
   B. early in the evening.
   C. after eating a full meal.
   D. when you feel most alert.

Answer: D. Study when you're most alert. If you feel most alert and energized in the morning, for example, set aside sections of time in the morning for topics that need a lot of review.

2. The temperature of the ideal study area should be between:
   A. 60° and 65° F.
   B. 65° and 70° F.
   C. 70° and 75° F.
   D. 75° and 80° F.

Answer: B. The ideal study area has a temperature between 65° and 70° F.

3. To help you maintain concentration during long study periods, recommended study strategies include:
   A. Study the topics you find most interesting first, followed by the topics you find least interesting.
   B. Study the topics you find least interesting first, followed by the topics you find most interesting.
   C. Alternate the order of the subjects you study during the day.
   D. Study only the topics you find least interesting; you'll remember the others.

Answer: C. Alternating the order of the subjects you study during the day adds variety to your study and helps you remain focused and make the most of your study time.

4. When selecting a study partner, choose one who:
   A. possesses similar goals as you.
   B. is highly social and will keep you entertained.
   C. isn't as knowledgeable as you so you can tutor him.
   D. likes to take a lot of breaks.

Answer: A. A partner who doesn't fit your needs won't help you make the most of your study time. Look for a partner who has similar goals to yours, possesses about the same level of knowledge as you, and won't spend too much time socializing.

Scoring

☆☆☆   If you answered all four questions correctly, wow! We hope the exam is ready for *you!*

☆☆   If you answered three questions correctly, terrific! You're cruising toward an exam day victory!

☆   If you answered fewer than three questions correctly, fear not. By the time you're done practicing, you'll be an NCLEX success!

Part II   Comprehensive tests

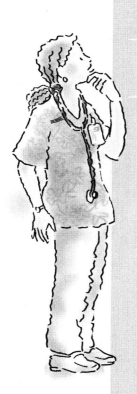

Comprehensive test 1   **33**

Comprehensive test 2   **52**

Comprehensive test 3   **70**

Comprehensive test 4   **89**

Comprehensive test 5   **109**

Comprehensive test 6   **128**

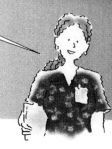

This comprehensive test, the first of six, is just like a real NCLEX test. It's a great way to practice!

COMPREHENSIVE
Test 1

1. A 43-year-old client with blunt chest trauma from a motor vehicle collision has sinus tachycardia, is hypotensive, and has developed muffled heart sounds. There are no obvious signs of bleeding. Which condition is suspected?
   1. Heart failure
   2. Pneumothorax
   3. Cardiac tamponade
   4. Myocardial infarction (MI)

2. The client is experiencing tamponade. Which type of shock should the nurse expect to observe in the client?
   1. Anaphylactic
   2. Cardiogenic
   3. Hypovolemic
   4. Septic

3. A nurse asks a nursing assistant to help admit an elderly client diagnosed with pneumonia. Which activity is appropriate for the nurse to ask the assistant to perform?
   1. Obtain the client's height and weight.
   2. Obtain an arterial blood gas sample.
   3. Insert a small-bore feeding tube.
   4. Assess lung sounds.

1. 3. Cardiac tamponade results in signs of obvious shock and muffled heart sounds. Heart failure would result in inspiratory crackles, pulmonary edema, and jugular vein distention. Pneumothorax would result in diminished breath sounds in the affected lung, respiratory distress, and tracheal displacement. In an MI, the client may complain of chest pain. Also, an electrocardiogram could confirm changes consistent with an MI.
CN: Physiological integrity; CNS: Physiological adaptation; CL: Analysis

2. 2. Fluid accumulates in the pericardial sac, hindering motion of the heart muscle and causing it to pump inefficiently, resulting in signs of cardiogenic shock. Anaphylactic and septic are types of distributive shock in which fluid is displaced from the capillaries and leaks into surrounding tissues. Hypovolemic shock involves the actual loss of fluid.
CN: Physiological integrity; CNS: Physiological adaptation; CL: Application

3. 1. Obtaining the client's height and weight are appropriate actions for the nursing assistant to perform. The other options are the responsibility of the registered nurse or other licensed person.
CN: Safe effective care environment; CNS: Management of care; CL: Application

CN: Client needs category   CNS: Client needs subcategory   TL: Cognitive level

4. The client is experiencing cardiac tamponade. Which intervention or medication should the nurse expect to see prescribed as the most appropriate treatment for this client?
1. Surgery
2. Dopamine
3. Blood transfusion
4. Pericardiocentesis

5. A nurse is teaching a 50-year-old client how to decrease risk factors for coronary artery disease. He's an executive who smokes, has a type A personality, and is hypertensive. Which risk factor is nonmodifiable?
1. Age
2. Hypertension
3. Personality
4. Smoking

6. A client says he's stressed by his job but enjoys the challenge. Which suggestion is best to help the client?
1. Switch job positions.
2. Take stress management classes.
3. Spend more time with his family.
4. Avoid working from home.

7. A nurse is teaching a client with glaucoma the proper technique for instilling eyedrops. She instructs the client to place the drops:
1. on the cornea.
2. in the outer canthus.
3. near the opening of the lacrimal duct.
4. in the lower conjunctival sac.

4. 4. Pericardiocentesis, or needle aspiration of the pericardial cavity, is done to relieve tamponade. An opening is created surgically if the client continues to have recurrent episodes of tamponade. Dopamine is used to restore blood pressure in normovolemic individuals. Blood transfusions may be given if the client is hypovolemic from blood loss.
CN: Physiological integrity; CNS: Physiological adaptation; CL: Application

5. 1. Age is a risk factor that is nonmodifiable. Type A personality, hypertension, and smoking factors can be controlled.
CN: Health promotion and maintenance; CNS: None; CL: Application

6. 2. Stress management classes will teach the client how to better manage the stress in his life, after identifying the factors that contribute to it. Alternatives may be found to leaving his job, which he enjoys. Not spending enough time with his family and taking his job home with him haven't yet been identified as contributing factors.
CN: Physiological integrity; CNS: Reduction of risk potential; CL: Application

7. 4. Eyedrops should be placed in the lower conjunctival sac starting at the inner, not outer canthus. Placing eyedrops on the cornea causes discomfort and should be avoided. Eyedrops shouldn't be placed by the opening of the lacrimal ducts to avoid systemic absorption.
CN: Physiological integrity; CNS: Pharmacological and parenteral therapies; CL: Application

CN: Client needs category   CNS: Client needs subcategory   CL: Cognitive level

8. A 28-year-old client with human immunodeficiency virus (HIV) is admitted to the hospital with flulike symptoms. He has dyspnea and a cough. He's placed on a 100% nonrebreather mask and arterial blood gases are drawn. Which result indicates the need for intubation?
1. Pa_{O_2}, 90 mm Hg; Pa_{CO_2}, 40 mm Hg
2. Pa_{O_2}, 85 mm Hg; Pa_{CO_2}, 45 mm Hg
3. Pa_{O_2}, 80 mm Hg; Pa_{CO_2}, 45 mm Hg
4. Pa_{O_2}, 70 mm Hg; Pa_{CO_2}, 55 mm Hg

9. The nurse is instructing a client regarding transmission of human immunodeficiency virus (HIV). What should the nurse instruct the client as to the most likely route of the virus' transmission?
1. Blood
2. Feces
3. Saliva
4. Urine

10. A client with acquired immunodeficiency syndrome has developed a protozoa infection. Which opportunistic infection will the client be most likely to develop as a result of the protozoa infection?
1. Tuberculosis (TB)
2. Histoplasmosis
3. Kaposi's sarcoma
4. *Pneumocystis jiroveci* infection

11. A client with acquired immunodeficiency syndrome is intubated, leaving him prone to skin breakdown from the endotracheal (ET) tube. Which intervention is best to prevent this?
1. Use lubricant on the lips.
2. Provide oral care every 2 hours.
3. Suction the oral cavity every 2 hours.
4. Reposition the ET tube every 24 hours.

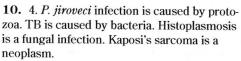

Ten questions done! Are you having fun yet?

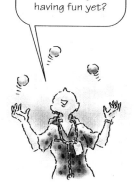

8. 4. An increasing Pa_{CO_2} and decreasing Pa_{O_2} indicate poor oxygen perfusion. Normal Pa_{O_2} levels are 80 to 100 mm Hg and normal Pa_{CO_2} levels are 35 to 45 mm Hg.
CN: Physiological integrity; CNS: Reduction of risk potential; CL: Analysis

9. 1. HIV is transmitted by contact with infected blood. It exists in all body fluids but transmission through saliva, urine, and feces is much less likely to occur than through blood.
CN: Safe, effective care environment; CNS: Safety and infection control; CL: Application

10. 4. *P. jiroveci* infection is caused by protozoa. TB is caused by bacteria. Histoplasmosis is a fungal infection. Kaposi's sarcoma is a neoplasm.
CN: Physiological integrity; CNS: Physiological adaptation; CL: Application

11. 4. Pressure causes skin breakdown. However, repositioning the ET tube from one side of the mouth to the other or to the center of the mouth can relieve pressure in one area for a time. Extreme care must be taken to move the tube only laterally; it must not be pushed in or pulled out. The tape securing the tube must be changed daily. Two nurses should perform this procedure. Oral care, suctioning, and lubricant help keep skin clean and intact and reduce the risk of further infection.
CN: Physiological integrity; CNS: Basic care and comfort; CL: Application

12. A client with acquired immunodeficiency syndrome has developed *Pneumocystis carinii* pneumonia and has begun treatment with pentamidine isethionate (Pentam). Based on the diagnosis and treatment, which medication is most likely to be ordered for the client?
   1. Amphotericin B
   2. Co-trimoxazole (Bactrim)
   3. Fluconazole (Diflucan)
   4. Sulfadiazine

13. A client is receiving pentamidine isethionate (Pentam). Which parameter will the nurse monitor frequently while the client receives this medication?
   1. Heart rate
   2. Electrolyte levels
   3. Blood sugar levels
   4. Complete blood count (CBC)

14. A nurse caring for a client with acquired immunodeficiency syndrome is working with a nursing student. She notes the student doesn't attempt to suction or assist with care of the client. Which action is appropriate?
   1. Talk to the student.
   2. Talk to the charge nurse.
   3. Address a coworker with the concerns.
   4. Seek advice from the student's instructor.

15. A client's significant other is tearful over the client's condition and lack of improvement. He says he feels powerless and unable to help his friend. Which response by the nurse is the best?
   1. Agree with the person.
   2. Tell him there's nothing he can do.
   3. State she understands how he must feel.
   4. Ask if he would like to help with some comfort measures.

12. 2. Co-trimoxazole is given orally or I.V. for *P. carinii* pneumonia. Fluconazole and amphotericin B are used for coccidioidomycosis. Sulfadiazine is used to treat toxoplasmosis.
CN: Physiological integrity; CNS: Pharmacological and parenteral therapies; CL: Application

13. 3. Pentamidine isethionate can cause permanent diabetes mellitus and requires monitoring of blood sugar levels. The client's electrolyte levels, heart rate, and CBC can be monitored less frequently.
CN: Physiological integrity; CNS: Pharmacological and parenteral therapies; CL: Application

14. 1. The nurse should approach the student to determine her feelings and experience in caring for this client. The charge nurse and coworkers aren't familiar with the student's abilities, but the instructor may be approached if the nurse can't communicate with the student.
CN: Safe, effective care environment; CNS: Management of care; CL: Analysis

15. 4. The significant other expresses a need to help and the nurse can encourage him to do whatever he feels comfortable with, such as putting lubricant on lips, moist cloth on forehead, or lotion on skin. The nurse may not understand his situation, and agreeing with a person doesn't diminish powerlessness. There are many ways the significant other can help if he wants to.
CN: Psychosocial integrity; CNS: None; CL: Analysis

CN: Client needs category   CNS: Client needs subcategory   CL: Cognitive level

16. A 31-year-old client is admitted to the hospital with respiratory failure. He's intubated in the emergency department, placed on 100% FIO_2, and is coughing up copious secretions. Which intervention should be done first?
1. Get an X-ray.
2. Suction the client.
3. Restrain the client.
4. Obtain an arterial blood gas (ABG) analysis.

17. A client with an endotracheal (ET) tube has copious, brown-tinged secretions. Which intervention is a priority?
1. Use a trap to obtain a specimen.
2. Instill saline to break up secretions.
3. Culture the specimen with a culturette swab.
4. Obtain an order for a liquefying agent for the sputum.

18. An X-ray shows an endotracheal (ET) tube is 2 cm above the carina, and there are nodular lesions and patchy infiltrates in the upper lobe. Which interpretation of the X-ray is accurate?
1. The X-ray is inconclusive.
2. The client has a disease process going on.
3. The ET tube needs to be advanced.
4. The ET tube needs to be pulled back.

19. A client has copious secretions. X-ray results indicate tuberculosis (TB). For which intervention should the nurse prepare the client first?
1. Repeat X-ray
2. Tracheostomy
3. Bronchoscopy
4. Arterial blood gas (ABG) analysis

16. 2. Secretions can cut off the oxygen supply to the client and result in hypoxia so suctioning the client is your first priority. X-rays are a priority to check placement of the endotracheal tube. Restraints are warranted if the client is a threat to his safety. After the client has acclimated to his ventilator settings, ABGs can be drawn.
CN: Physiological integrity; CNS: Reduction of risk potential; CL: Analysis

17. 1. Suspicious secretions should be sent for culture and sensitivity using a sterile technique such as a trap. Saline would dilute the specimen. Swab culturettes are useful for wound cultures — not ET cultures. Various agents are available to help break up secretions, and respiratory therapists can usually help recommend the right agent, but this isn't a priority.
CN: Safe, effective care environment; CNS: Safety and infection control; CL: Analysis

18. 2. The X-ray is suggestive of tuberculosis. At 2 cm, the ET tube is at an adequate level in the trachea and doesn't have to be advanced or pulled back.
CN: Physiological integrity; CNS: Reduction of risk potential; CL: Analysis

19. 3. Bronchoscopy can help diagnose TB and obtain specimens while clearing the bronchial tree of secretions. X-rays may be repeated periodically to determine lung and endotracheal tube status. Tracheostomy may be done if the client remains on the ventilator for a prolonged period. A change in condition or treatment may require an ABG analysis.
CN: Physiological integrity; CNS: Reduction of risk potential; CL: Application

20. A nurse is aware that family members of a client diagnosed with tuberculosis may have been exposed to the disease. The nurse explains that a tuberculin skin test should be performed on each family member and that this may show:
1. active disease.
2. recent infection.
3. extent of the infection.
4. infection at some point.

21. A client is diagnosed with tuberculosis (TB). In addition to recommending skin testing of the family members, TB should be reported to which individual or agency?
1. Centers for Disease Control and Prevention (CDC)
2. Local health department
3. Infection-control nurse
4. Client's physician

22. A client with tuberculosis (TB) is being treated with isoniazid (INH). Which therapy is most likely to be ordered in conjunction with INH?
1. Theophylline inhaler
2. I.M. penicillin
3. Multiple antibacterial agents
4. Aerosol treatments with pentamidine (Pentam)

23. A nurse is teaching a client with tuberculosis (TB) about his medication treatment. She should explain that most clients receive treatment for TB for:
1. 2 to 4 months.
2. 9 to 12 months.
3. 18 to 24 months.
4. more than 2 years.

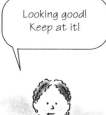

Looking good! Keep at it!

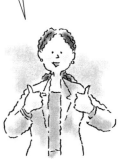

20. 4. A tuberculin skin test shows the presence of infection at some point; a positive skin test doesn't guarantee that an infection is *currently* present, however. Some people have false-positive results. Active disease may be viewed on a chest X-ray. Computed tomography or magnetic resonance imaging can evaluate the extent of lung damage.

CN: Safe, effective care environment; CNS: Safety and infection control; CL: Application

21. 2. The local health department must be informed of an outbreak of TB because it's a reportable disease. They, in turn, inform the CDC. The infection-control nurse or employee health department may request that staff be tested if exposed. Generally, the client's family can inform his physician.

CN: Safe, effective care environment; CNS: Safety and infection control; CL: Application

22. 3. Because TB has become resistant to many antibacterial agents, the initial treatment includes the use of multiple antituberculotic or antibacterial drugs. These may include rifampin, ethambutol hydrochloride, pyrazinamide, cycloserine, clofazimine, and streptomycin. Theophylline is a bronchodilator used to treat asthma and chronic obstructive pulmonary disease. Penicillins are used to treat *Staphylococcus aureus*—not TB. Pentamidine is used in the treatment of pneumonia caused by *Pneumocystis jiroveci*.

CN: Physiological integrity; CNS: Pharmacological and parenteral therapies; CL: Application

23. 2. Treatment for TB is usually continued for at least 9 to 12 months.

CN: Physiological integrity; CNS: Pharmacological and parenteral therapies; CL: Application

CN: Client needs category CNS: Client needs subcategory CL: Cognitive level

24. A nurse teaches a client with tuberculosis that he is still considered infectious after treatment is started for which period of time?
   1. 72 hours
   2. 1 week
   3. 2 weeks
   4. 4 weeks

25. A client tells his nurse that his tuberculosis medications are so expensive that he can't afford to take them. Which intervention by the nurse is best?
   1. Refer the client to social services.
   2. Tell the client to apply for Medicaid.
   3. Refer the client to the local or county health department.
   4. Tell the client to follow his insurance rules and regulations.

26. A 62-year-old client is admitted to the hospital with pneumonia. He has a history of Parkinson's disease, which his family says is progressively worsening. Which assessment is expected?
   1. Impaired speech
   2. Muscle flaccidity
   3. Pleasant and smiling demeanor
   4. Tremors in the fingers that increase with purposeful movement

27. Which nursing diagnosis describes a clinical judgment that an individual, family, or community is more vulnerable to developing a certain problem than others in the same or similar situation are?
   1. *Risk for compromised human dignity*
   2. *Moral distress*
   3. *Stress overload*
   4. *Readiness for enhanced comfort*

24. 4. After 4 weeks, the disease is no longer infectious but the client must continue to take the medication.

CN: Safe, effective care environment; CNS: Safety and infection control; CL: Application

25. 3. The local and county health departments provide treatment and follow-up free of charge for all residents to ensure proper care. Social services can help seek alternative methods of payment and reimbursement but would probably first refer the client to the local and county health departments. Medicaid or medical assistance is another avenue for the client, *if* he qualifies. Insurance can be an alternative source to help pay for treatment, but the client may not be insured or the policy may not cover prescriptions.

CN: Safe, effective care environment; CNS: Management of care; CL: Analysis

26. 1. In Parkinson's disease, dysarthria, or impaired speech, is due to a disturbance in muscle control. Muscle rigidity results in resistance to passive muscle stretching. The client may have a masklike appearance. Tremors should decrease with purposeful movement and sleep.

CN: Physiological integrity; CNS: Physiological adaptation; CL: Application

27. 1. *Risk for compromised human dignity* is a risk nursing diagnosis that refers to the vulnerability of a client, family, or community to health problems. *Moral distress* and *Stress overload* are nursing diagnoses that describe a human response to a health problem being manifested. *Readiness for enhanced comfort* is a diagnostic statement describing the human response to levels of wellness in an individual, family, or community that have a potential for enhancement to a higher state.

CN: Safe, effective care environment; CNS: Management of care; CL: Analysis

28. A client is ordered to receive 1,000 ml of 0.45% normal saline with 20 mEq of potassium chloride (KCL) over 6 hours. The infusion set administers 15 gtt/ml. At how many gtt/minute should the nurse set the flow rate?
 1. 36
 2. 40
 3. 42
 4. 45

28. 3. The flow rate is determined by the rate of infusion and the number of drops per milliliters of the fluid being administered:
gtt/ml × amount to be infused divided by the number of minutes = the intravenous flow rate.
$15 \text{ gtt/ml} \times 1000 \text{ ml} = 15,000$
$15,000 \text{ ml} \div 360 \text{ minutes} = 41.6 \text{ gtt/minute}$
Therefore, the flow rate should be 42 gtt/minute.
CN: Physiological integrity; CNS: Pharmacological and parenteral therapy; CL: Application

29. An 82-year-old male client with Parkinson's disease is frequently incontinent of urine. Which intervention should be done first?
 1. Diaper the client.
 2. Apply a condom catheter.
 3. Insert an indwelling urinary catheter.
 4. Provide skin care every 4 hours.

29. 2. A condom catheter uses a condom-type device to drain urine away from the client. Diapering the client may keep urine away from the body but may also be demeaning if the client is alert or the family objects. Because the client with Parkinson's disease is already prone to urinary tract infections, an indwelling urinary catheter should be avoided because it may promote this. Skin care must be provided as soon as the client is incontinent to prevent skin maceration and breakdown.
CN: Physiological integrity; CNS: Basic care and comfort; CL: Analysis

30. Family members report exhaustion and difficulty taking care of a dependent family member. Which approach is in the best interest of the client?
 1. Ask the client what he wishes.
 2. Have the family members discuss it among themselves.
 3. Tell the family the client should go to a nursing care facility.
 4. Call a family conference and ask social services for assistance.

30. 4. A family conference with social services can enlighten the family to all prospects of care available to them. The client should supply input if he's able but this may not help solve the problems of exhaustion and care difficulties. The family may not be aware of alternative care measures for the client, so a discussion among themselves may not be helpful. The client may not qualify for a nursing care facility because of stringent criteria.
CN: Safe, effective care environment; CNS: Management of care; CL: Analysis

31. A 30-year-old primagravida in her second trimester tells a nurse her fingers feel tight and sometimes she feels as though her heart skips a beat. She has a history of rheumatic fever. Which assessment indicates the client may be experiencing cardiovascular disease?
 1. Clear lungs
 2. Sinus tachycardia
 3. Increased dyspnea on exertion
 4. Runs of paroxysmal atrial tachycardia

31. 3. Increasing dyspnea on exertion should alert the nurse to cardiovascular compromise. Cardiac arrhythmias (other than sinus tachycardia or paroxysmal atrial tachycardia) and persistent crackles at the bases are also symptoms of cardiovascular disease.
CN: Health promotion and maintenance; CNS: None; CL: Analysis

CN: Client needs category CNS: Client needs subcategory CL: Cognitive level

32. Which diagnostic test may be performed to determine the extent of cardiovascular disease during pregnancy?
1. Stress test
2. Chest X-ray
3. Echocardiography
4. Cardiac catheterization

33. A 25-year-old primagravida has been in labor for 20 hours with little progress. The doctor prescribes oxytocin for her. The order reads 10 U oxytocin in 1,000 ml/NSS to infuse via pump at 1 mU/minute for 15 minutes; then increase flow rate to 2 mU/minute. What's the flow rate needed to deliver 1 mU/minute for 15 minutes?
1. 4 ml/hr
2. 6 ml/hr
3. 12 ml/hr
4. 16 ml/hr

34. Which statement by the nurse most accurately reflects subjective data in a nursing assessment?
1. "The client's red blood cell count is elevated."
2. "The client has a positive Babinski sign."
3. "The client's X-ray result showed a fracture present."
4. "The client reported that his pain is a 7 on a 1–10 scale."

35. Which classification of medication may be used safely in a pregnant client with cardiovascular disease?
1. Antibiotics
2. Warfarin (Coumadin)
3. Cardiac glycosides
4. Diuretics

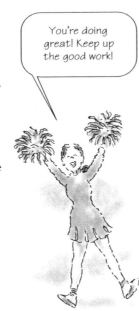

You're doing great! Keep up the good work!

32. 3. Echocardiography is less invasive than X-rays and other methods and provides the information needed to determine cardiovascular disease, especially valvular disorders. Cardiac catheterization and stress tests may be postponed until after delivery.
CN: Physiological integrity; CNS: Physiological adaptation; CL: Analysis

33. 2. First, determine the concentration of the solution with 10 U/1,000 ml as the known factor and X as the unknown factor:

$$\frac{10\ U}{1,000\ ml} = \frac{X}{1\ ml} \quad X = .01\ U/ml$$

Then, cross-multiply and solve for X. Next, convert to mU by multiplying by 1,000.

$$.01 \times 1,000 = 10\ mU/ml$$

Determine flow rate using the following equation:

$$\frac{10\ mU}{1\ ml} = \frac{15mU}{X} \quad X = \frac{15mU}{10} = 1.5\ ml$$

Convert to an hourly rate by multiplying by 4 (60 minutes/15 minutes = 4)

$$1.5\ ml/15\ minutes \times 4 = 6\ ml/hr$$

CN: Physiological integrity; CNS: Pharmacological and parenteral therapies; CL: Application

34. 4. Subjective data, also known as *symptoms* or *covert cues,* include the client's own verbatim statements about the health problems. Laboratory study results, physical assessment data, and diagnostic procedure reports are observable, perceptible, and measurable and can be verified and validated by others.
CN: Safe, effective care environment; CNS: Management of care; CL: Application

35. 3. Cardiac glycosides and common antiarrhythmics, such as procainamide (Procanbid) and quinidine (Quinaglute), may be used. Prophylactic antibiotics are reserved for clients susceptible to endocarditis. If anticoagulants are needed, heparin is the drug of choice—not warfarin. Diuretics should be used with extreme caution, if at all, because of the potential for causing uterine contractions.
CN: Physiological integrity; CNS: Pharmacological and parenteral therapies; CL: Analysis

36. A client arrives at the emergency department in her third trimester with painless vaginal bleeding. Which condition is suspected?
1. Placenta previa
2. Preterm labor
3. Abruptio placentae
4. A sexually transmitted infection (STI)

37. After assessing vital signs and applying an external monitor, which intervention is a priority for a client with suspected placenta previa?
1. Insert an indwelling urinary catheter.
2. Plan for an immediate cesarean delivery.
3. Place the client in Trendelenburg position.
4. Obtain blood work and start I.V. catheters.

38. A pregnant client with vaginal bleeding asks a nurse how the fetus is doing. Which is the best response for the nurse to give?
1. "I don't know for sure."
2. "I can't answer that question."
3. "It's too early to tell anything."
4. "Here's what the monitor shows."

39. A client is hospitalized at 35 weeks' gestation with placenta previa and placed on strict bedrest. She states "I lost my last baby at 24 weeks." Which nursing diagnosis would the nurse set as the priority?
1. *Risk for constipation related to immobility*
2. *Anxiety related to unknown fetal outcome*
3. *Impaired physical mobility related to bedrest*
4. *Ineffective coping related to inappropriate thinking*

40. A neonate requires blood transfusions after birth. Which cannulation site is most preferred?
1. Scalp veins
2. Intraosseous
3. Umbilical cord
4. Subclavian cutdown

36. 1. Placenta previa presents with painless vaginal bleeding. Abruptio placentae usually includes vague abdominal discomfort and tenderness. Preterm labor and STIs usually don't cause bleeding.
CN: Health promotion and maintenance; CNS: None; CL: Analysis

37. 4. Blood for hemoglobin, hematocrit, type, and crossmatch should be collected and I.V. catheters inserted. The nurse shouldn't attempt Trendelenburg positioning or urinary catheterization. The client may be placed on her left side. Depending on the degree of bleeding and fetal maturity, a cesarean delivery may be required.
CN: Physiological integrity; CNS: Reduction of risk potential; CL: Application

38. 4. The client deserves a truthful answer and the nurse should be objective without giving opinions. Vague answers may be misleading and aren't therapeutic.
CN: Psychosocial integrity; CNS: None; CL: Analysis

39. 2. The client's statement reflects concern for her fetus. Therefore the priority diagnosis is *Anxiety related to unknown fetal outcome.* The client may be at risk for constipation and mobility is impaired but these aren't the priority. There's no indication of a disturbed thought process.
CN: Safe, effective care environment; CNS: Management of care; CL: Analysis

40. 3. The umbilical cord may be easily cannulated and is the preferred site. Scalp veins may also be used. Intraosseous cannulation is attempted if two attempts at other sites prove inaccessible. A subclavian cutdown takes a prolonged time and is the least desired.
CN: Health promotion and maintenance; CNS: None; CL: Analysis

41. A nurse working in the triage area of an emergency department sees that several pediatric clients arrive simultaneously. Which client should be treated first?
1. A crying 4-year-old child with a laceration on his scalp
2. A 3-year-old child with a barking cough and flushed appearance
3. A 3-year-old child with Down syndrome who's pale and asleep in his mother's arms
4. A 2-year-old child with stridorous breath sounds, sitting up in his mother's arms and drooling

42. A 2-year-old child is being examined in the emergency department for epiglottitis. Which assessment finding supports this diagnosis?
1. Mild fever
2. Clear speech
3. Tripod position
4. Gradual onset of symptoms

43. Which method is best when approaching a 2-year-old child to listen to breath sounds?
1. Tell the child it's time to listen to his lungs now.
2. Tell the child to lie down while the nurse listens to his lungs.
3. Ask the caregiver to wait outside while the nurse listens to his lungs.
4. Ask if he would like the nurse to listen to the front or the back of his chest first.

44. A mother says that her 2-year-old child is up to date with his immunizations. The nurse can most accurately determine that the client is up-to-date with his immunizations if his immunizations included:
1. Diptheria-pertussis-tetanus (DTaP), inactivated polio (IPV), measles-mumps-rubella (MMR)
2. DTaP, IPV, MMR, Hemophilus influenza type B (Hib), varicella, pneumococcal, hepatitis B, Rotavirus (Rota)
3. DTaP, hepatitis B, IPV
4. MMR, IPV, hepatitis B

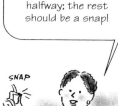

You're more than halfway; the rest should be a snap!

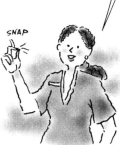

SNAP

41. 4. The infant with the airway emergency should be treated first, because of the risk of epiglottitis. The 3-year-old with the barking cough and fever should be suspected of having croup and should be seen promptly, as should the child with the laceration. The nurse would need to gather information about the child with Down syndrome to determine the priority of care.
CN: Safe, effective care environment; CNS: Management of care; CL: Analysis

42. 3. The tripod position (sitting up and leaning forward) facilitates breathing. Epiglottitis presents with a sudden onset of symptoms, high fever, and muffled speech. Additional symptoms are inspiratory stridor and drooling.
CN: Physiological integrity; CNS: Physiological adaptation; CL: Application

43. 4. The 2-year-old child needs to feel in control, and this approach best supports the child's independence. Giving the child no choice may make him uncooperative. The child should be allowed to remain in the tripod position to facilitate breathing. The caregiver should be allowed to remain with the child because fear of separation is common in 2-year-olds.
CN: Health promotion and maintenance; CNS: None; CL: Application

44. 2. By the age of 2, the DTaP, IPV, MMR, Hib, varicella, pneumococcal, hepatitis B and Rotavirus vaccines should have been received. The nurse should clarify this with the mother or caregiver.
CN: Safe, effective care environment; CNS: Safety and infection control; CL: Application

45. Which condition is the biggest threat for a child who has been diagnosed with epiglottitis?
1. Airway obstruction
2. Dehydration
3. Malnutrition
4. Seizures

46. What is the most accurate way of diagnosing epiglottitis?
1. Lateral neck X-ray
2. Direct visualization
3. History of sudden onset
4. Presenting signs and symptoms

47. A student nurse working with a registered nurse is assessing a child with epiglottitis. The student tells the client she needs to look at his throat. Which intervention by the registered nurse is best?
1. Hand her a flashlight and tongue blade.
2. Give her a sterile tongue blade and culturette swab.
3. Tell the student that the registered nurse will visualize the child's throat.
4. Tell the student visualization will be done by the anesthesiologist.

48. The mother of a 2-year-old child with epiglottitis says she needs to pick up her older child from school. The 2-year-old child begins to cry and appears more stridorous. Which intervention by the nurse is best?
1. Ask the mother how long she may be gone.
2. Tell the 2-year-old everything will be all right.
3. Tell the 2-year-old the nurse will stay with him.
4. Ask the mother if there's anyone else who can meet the older child.

45. 1. The biggest threat to the child is airway obstruction because of the inflammation and swelling of the epiglottis and surrounding tissue. Dehydration can be prevented with I.V. therapy and seizures averted by decreasing the fever. Malnutrition is least likely to occur because epiglottiditis is a short-lived situation.
CN: Physiological integrity; CNS: Reduction of risk potential; CL: Application

46. 4. The presenting symptoms are diagnostic of epiglottitis. Lateral neck X-rays aren't necessary. Only an anesthesiologist or physician skilled in intubation should do direct visualization. History of sudden onset helps support the assessment, but a history alone wouldn't be sufficient to make a diagnosis.
CN: Health promotion and maintenance; CNS: None; CL: Application

47. 4. Direct visualization of the epiglottis can trigger a complete airway obstruction and should only be done in a controlled environment by an anesthesiologist or a physician skilled in pediatric intubation.
CN: Safe, effective care environment; CNS: Management of care; CL: Application

48. 4. Increased anxiety and agitation should be avoided in the child to prevent airway obstruction. A 2-year-old child fears separation from parents, so the mother should be encouraged to stay. Other means of picking up the older child need to be found. Telling the child that everything will be all right may not decrease his agitation; the mother is the primary caregiver and important to the child for emotional and security reasons.
CN: Health promotion and maintenance; CNS: None; CL: Analysis

CN: Client needs category   CNS: Client needs subcategory   CL: Cognitive level

49. A father arrives in a busy emergency department and is upset with his wife for bringing their 2-year-old child with epiglottitis in for treatment. Which intervention by the nurse is best?
1. Leave the room.
2. Call for security.
3. Recognize the father's behavior as his attempt to cope with the situation.
4. Tell both parents to leave because they're upsetting the child.

50. A 40-year-old client is being treated for GI bleeding. On his fifth day of hospitalization, he begins to have tremors, is agitated, and is experiencing hallucinations. These signs suggest which condition?
1. Alcohol withdrawal
2. Allergic response
3. Alzheimer's disease
4. Hypoxia

51. If a nurse suspects a client is experiencing alcohol withdrawal syndrome, which action is appropriate?
1. Verify it with family.
2. Inform social services.
3. Ask the client about his drinking.
4. Tell the client everything will be all right.

52. A client experiencing alcohol withdrawal syndrome says he sees cockroaches on the ceiling. Which response is most appropriate?
1. Ask the client where he sees them.
2. Ask the client if the cockroaches are still there.
3. Tell the client there are no cockroaches on the ceiling.
4. Tell the client it's dim in the room and turn on the overhead lights.

49. 3. Lack of control over his son's situation results in irrational behavior. The nurse should try to calm both parents and let them know they did the right thing due to the seriousness of their child's situation. Calling for security, sending the parents out, or leaving the room won't help the child nor will it reduce frustration or inappropriate behavior.
CN: Safe, effective care environment; CNS: Management of care; CL: Analysis

50. 1. These are signs of alcohol withdrawal syndrome, which can begin 5 to 7 days after the last drink. An allergic reaction would cause difficulty breathing, skin rash, or edema as primary symptoms. Alzheimer's disease occurs in older individuals and has other psychosocial signs, such as a masklike face and altered mentation. Hypoxia would cause symptoms of respiratory distress.
CN: Psychosocial integrity; CNS: None; CL: Analysis

51. 3. Confirming suspicions with the client is the most beneficial way to help in diagnosis and treatment. If the client isn't cooperative, verification can be sought from the family. Social services aren't required at this time but may be helpful in discharge planning. Giving false reassurance isn't therapeutic for the client.
CN: Psychosocial integrity; CNS: None; CL: Application

52. 4. Try to reorient the client to reality and minimize distortions. Don't support the client's hallucinations or place the client on the defensive but try to present reality gently without agitating the client.
CN: Psychosocial integrity; CNS: None; CL: Application

53. A client experiencing alcohol withdrawal syndrome says he's itching everywhere from the bugs on his bed. Which response is appropriate?
1. Examine the client's skin.
2. Ask what kind of bugs he thinks they are.
3. Tell the client there are no bugs on his bed.
4. Tell the client he's having tactile hallucinations.

54. A client with alcohol withdrawal syndrome is pulling at his central venous catheter, saying he's swatting the spiders crawling over him. Which intervention is most appropriate?
1. Encourage the client to rest.
2. Protect the client from harm.
3. Tell the client there are no spiders.
4. Tell the client he's pulling the I.V. tubing.

55. A client who experienced alcohol withdrawal syndrome is no longer having hallucinations or tremors and says he would like to enter a rehabilitation facility to stop drinking. Which intervention is appropriate?
1. Ask about his insurance.
2. Tell him he should talk with his family.
3. Refer him to Alcoholics Anonymous (AA).
4. Promote participation in a treatment program.

56. A 72-year-old man with cirrhosis is admitted to the hospital in a hepatic coma. Based on his condition, which nursing intervention will have the highest priority?
1. Perform a neurologic check.
2. Complete the client admission.
3. Orient the client to his environment.
4. Check airway, breathing, and circulation.

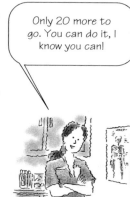

Only 20 more to go. You can do it, I know you can!

53. 1. Make sure the client doesn't have a rash, skin allergy, or something on his skin (such as crumbs) causing his discomfort. Reality should then be presented to the client gently without being derogatory. The nurse shouldn't support the client's hallucinations.
CN: Psychosocial integrity; CNS: None; CL: Application

54. 2. During periods of alcohol withdrawal syndrome, the client needs to be protected from harm. If the client dislodges the central venous catheter, he may incur an air embolus, which can be life-threatening. Although reality should be presented to the client, telling him that there are no spiders and that he's pulling the I.V. tubing may not make him stop; therefore, his safety is still at risk. The client may need to be restrained if continued observation during this time isn't available. The client should also be encouraged to rest; however, this intervention doesn't take priority over safety.
CN: Psychosocial integrity; CNS: None; CL: Analysis

55. 4. The client should be encouraged to enter a facility if that's in his best interest. Arrangements that are covered by his insurance can be made and discussed with the social service coordinator and his physician. The client can inform his family, and support should be encouraged. Referral to AA should be considered after rehabilitation takes place.
CN: Psychosocial integrity; CNS: None; CL: Application

56. 4. Priorities include airway, breathing, and circulation. Once these are ensured, a neurologic check is needed to determine status. General orientation and completing the admission may require the help and affirmation of family members. Depending on the client's alertness, orientation to the environment may need to be kept simple (where he is, date, time).
CN: Physiological integrity; CNS: Reduction of risk potential; CL: Application

CN: Client needs category CNS: Client needs subcategory CL: Cognitive level

57. A client with cirrhosis is restless and at times tries to climb out of bed. Which intervention is best to promote safety?
    1. Use leather restraints.
    2. Use soft wrist restraints.
    3. Use a vest restraint device.
    4. Use a sheet tied across the client's chest.

58. The nurse is assessing a client with cirrhosis. Which finding is most consistent with late-stage cirrhosis?
    1. Constipation
    2. Diarrhea
    3. Hypoxia
    4. Vomiting

59. A client with cirrhosis is jaundiced and edematous. He's experiencing severe itching and dryness. Which intervention is best to help the client?
    1. Put mitts on his hands.
    2. Use alcohol-free body lotion.
    3. Lubricate the skin with baby oil.
    4. Wash the skin with soap and water.

60. A 20-year-old client with a spinal cord injury sustained in a previous motorcycle collision is hospitalized for renal calculi, or kidney stones. To reduce the client's risk for developing recurrent kidney stones, which instruction is correct?
    1. Eat yogurt daily.
    2. Drink cranberry juice.
    3. Eat more fresh fruits and vegetables.
    4. Increase the intake of dairy products.

61. A client with a spinal cord injury says he has difficulty recognizing the symptoms of urinary tract infection (UTI) before it's too late. Which symptom is an early sign of UTI?
    1. Lower back pain
    2. Burning on urination
    3. Frequency of urination
    4. Fever and change in the clarity of urine

57. 3. The client may require gentle reminders not to get out of bed to prevent a fall. The vest restraint would help in this endeavor. Leather restraints are only warranted for extremely combative and unsafe clients. Soft wrist restraints may not stop the client from sitting up or trying to swing his legs over the bed rails. A sheet tied across the client's chest can hamper breathing or may asphyxiate the client if he slides down in the bed.
CN: Safe, effective care environment; CNS: Management of care; CL: Analysis

58. 3. In late-stage cirrhosis, fluid in the lungs and weak chest expansion can lead to hypoxia. Diarrhea, vomiting, and constipation are early signs and symptoms of cirrhosis.
CN: Physiological integrity; CNS: Physiological adaptation; CL: Application

59. 2. Alcohol-free body lotion applied to the skin can help relieve dryness and is absorbed without oiliness. Mitts may help keep the client from scratching his skin open. Soap dries out the skin. Baby oil doesn't allow excretions through the skin and may block pores.
CN: Physiological integrity; CNS: Basic care and comfort; CL: Application

60. 2. Acid urine decreases the potential for kidney stones. The majority of renal calculi form in alkaline urine. Cranberries, prunes, and plums promote acidic urine. Yogurt helps restore pH balance to secretions in yeast infections. Fruits and vegetables increase fiber in the diet and promote alkaline urine. Dairy products may contribute to the formation of kidney stones.
CN: Physiological integrity; CNS: Reduction of risk potential; CL: Application

61. 4. The client with a spinal cord injury should recognize fever and change in the clarity of urine as early signs of UTI. Lower back pain is a late sign. The client with a spinal cord injury may not have burning or frequency of urination.
CN: Physiological integrity; CNS: Reduction of risk potential; CL: Application

62. A client tells a nurse he boils his urinary catheters to keep them sterile. Which question should the nurse ask the client?
1. "What technique is used for catheterization?"
2. "At what temperature are the catheters boiled?"
3. "Why aren't prepackaged sterile catheters used?"
4. "Are the catheters dried and stored in a clean, dry place?"

63. A 60-year-old client had a colostomy 4 days ago due to rectal cancer and is having trouble adjusting to it. Which nursing diagnosis would be the most common for the client following this procedure?
1. *Anxiety*
2. *Situational low self-esteem*
3. *Impaired comfort*
4. *Disturbed body image*

64. A nurse approaches a client with a recent colostomy for a routine assessment and finds him tearful. Which action is appropriate?
1. State she'll come back another time.
2. Ask the client if he's having pain or discomfort.
3. Tell the client she needs to perform an assessment.
4. Sit down with the client and ask if he'd like to talk about anything.

65. After a review of colostomy care, a client says he doesn't know if he'll be able to care for himself at home without help. Which nursing intervention is most appropriate to ensure continuity of care?
1. Review care with the client again.
2. Provide written instructions for the client.
3. Ask the client if there's anyone who can help.
4. Arrange for home health care to visit the client.

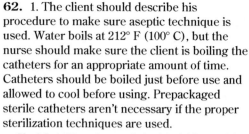
You're almost finished. Keep pluggin' away!

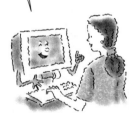

62. 1. The client should describe his procedure to make sure aseptic technique is used. Water boils at 212° F (100° C), but the nurse should make sure the client is boiling the catheters for an appropriate amount of time. Catheters should be boiled just before use and allowed to cool before using. Prepackaged sterile catheters aren't necessary if the proper sterilization techniques are used.
CN: Physiological integrity; CNS: Reduction of risk potential; CL: Analysis

63. 4. *Disturbed body image* is most common with a new colostomy and dealing with its care. The client shouldn't have signs of anxiety but he may not be comfortable caring for the colostomy. Low self-esteem may also be a concern for the client, but may not be as common as disturbed body image. The client should be having less discomfort postoperatively.
CN: Safe, effective care environment; CNS: Management of care; CL: Application

64. 4. Asking open-ended questions and appearing interested in what the client has to say will encourage verbalization of feelings. Leaving the client may make him feel unaccepted. Asking closed-ended questions won't encourage verbalization of feelings. Ignoring the client's present state isn't therapeutic for the client.
CN: Psychosocial integrity; CNS: None; CL: Application

65. 4. Although all of these interventions may benefit the patient, arranging for home health care will best ensure continuity of care.
CN: Safe, effective care environment; CNS: Management of care; CL: Application

CN: Client needs category CNS: Client needs subcategory CL: Cognitive level

66. A client is experiencing mild diarrhea through his colostomy. Which instruction is correct to give this client?
1. Eat prunes.
2. Drink apple juice.
3. Increase lettuce intake.
4. Increase intake of bananas.

67. A client reports a lot of gas in his colostomy bag. Which instruction is best to give this client?
1. Burp the bag.
2. Replace the bag.
3. Put a tiny hole in the top of the bag.
4. Eat less beans.

68. A client at a routine blood glucose screening for diabetes mellitus tells a nurse he has excessive urination and excessive thirst. The nurse should ask about which symptom first?
1. Weakness
2. Weight loss
3. Vision changes
4. Excessive hunger

69. A client recently diagnosed with pre-diabetes asks the nurse about the risk factors for developing diabetes mellitus. The nurse identifies which factor as the client's greatest risk for developing diabetes mellitus?
1. Obesity
2. Japanese descent
3. A great-grandparent with diabetes mellitus
4. Delivery of a neonate weighing more than 10 pounds

70. A 52-year-old client had gastric bypass surgery, is on nothing-by-mouth (NPO) status, and is in pain. The nurse gives meperidine (Demerol) 75 mg I.M. as ordered. In 20 minutes, he's feeling nauseous. What would the nurse suspect as the most likely cause?
1. The surgery is causing his nausea.
2. Because he's NPO, the increase in gastric secretions is precipitating this symptom.
3. Meperidine, which was given for his pain, has a tendency to cause nausea.
4. He may be reacting to blood still remaining in his mouth after extubation.

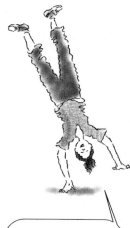

Five more to go! Oooooh, I'm getting excited!

66. 4. Bananas help make formed stool and aren't irritating to the bowel. Apple juice and prunes can increase the frequency of diarrhea. Lettuce acts as a fiber and can increase the looseness of stools.
CN: Physiological integrity; CNS: Basic care and comfort; CL: Application

67. 1. Letting air out of the bag by opening it and burping it is the best solution. Replacing the bag is costly. Putting a hole in the bag will also cause fluids to leak out. The client can be encouraged to note which foods are causing gas and to eat less gas-forming foods.
CN: Physiological integrity; CNS: Basic care and comfort; CL: Application

68. 4. Polyuria, polydipsia, and polyphagia are the three hallmark signs of diabetes mellitus. Weight loss, weakness, and vision changes also occur with diabetes mellitus.
CN: Health promotion and maintenance; CNS: None; CL: Application

69. 1. Obesity is a risk factor associated with diabetes mellitus. Delivery of a neonate weighing more than 9 lb, a family history of diabetes mellitus (mother, father, or sibling), and those of Native American, Black, Asian, or Hispanic descent are at high risk for developing diabetes mellitus, but obesity puts the client at greatest risk.
CN: Health promotion and maintenance; CNS: None; CL: Analysis

70. 3. Although gastric bypass surgery may precipitate some feelings of nausea, the timing of this symptom after the administration of meperidine is suspicious. Most likely, this client is experiencing a very common adverse effect of the analgesic meperidine. The status of being NPO wouldn't cause an increase in gastric secretions. It's possible that there may be some blood in his mouth after extubation, but the chances of this happening are minimal and less likely to be the cause of the client's complaint.
CN: Physiological integrity; CNS: Pharmacological and parenteral therapies; CL: Analysis

71. A client asks what diabetes mellitus does to the body over time. Which condition should the nurse include in her teaching as a common chronic complication of diabetes mellitus?
1. Multiple sclerosis
2. Diabetic ketoacidosis
3. Cardiovascular disease
4. Hyperosmolar hyperglycemic nonketotic syndrome (HHNS)

72. A client asks how he might decrease the risk of developing diabetes mellitus, which runs in his family. Which response is appropriate?
1. "Eat only poultry and fish."
2. "Omit carbohydrates from your diet."
3. "Start a moderate exercise program."
4. "Check blood glucose levels every month."

73. The nurse is assessing a client's arterial pulses. Which graphic displays the appropriate site for palpating the dorsalis pedis pulse?

1.

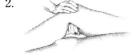

2.

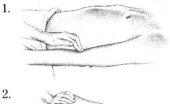

3.

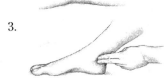

4.

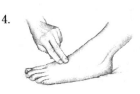

71. 3. Cardiovascular disease is a common chronic complication of diabetes mellitus. There's no known relationship between multiple sclerosis and diabetes mellitus. Diabetic ketoacidosis and HHNS are acute complications that can occur.
CN: Health promotion and maintenance; CNS: None; CL: Application

72. 3. Exercise and weight control are the goals in preventing and treating diabetes mellitus. Red meat can be eaten but should be limited because it contributes to cardiovascular disease. Complex carbohydrates account for a large portion of the diabetic diet and shouldn't be omitted. Checking blood glucose levels will help monitor the development of diabetes mellitus but won't prevent or decrease the chance of it occurring.
CN: Physiological integrity; CNS: Reduction of risk potential; CL: Application

73. 4. To palpate the dorsalis pedis pulse, the nurse places her fingers on the medial dorsum of the foot while the client points his toes down. The first graphic shows palpation of the brachial pulse. This pulse is palpated with the fingers placed medial to the biceps tendon. The second graphic shows palpation of the popliteal pulse in the popliteal fossa of the back of the knee. The third graphic shows palpation of the posterior tibial pulse, slightly below the malleolus of the ankle.
CN: Health promotion and maintenance; CNS: None; CL: Application

74. A nurse is having lunch in the hospital cafeteria when a visitor sitting at the next table begins to choke on his food. According to the American Heart Association (AHA), the nurse should intervene using the actions listed below. List the actions in the sequence in which she should perform them.

| 1. Administer abdominal thrusts until effective or until the client becomes unresponsive. |

| 2. Activate the emergency response team. |

| 3. Ask the client if he can speak. |

| 4. Start cardiopulmonary resuscitation (CPR). |

74.

| 3. Ask the client if he can speak. |

| 1. Administer abdominal thrusts until effective or until the client becomes unresponsive. |

| 2. Activate the emergency response team. |

| 4. Start cardiopulmonary resuscitation (CPR). |

According to the AHA, the nurse should ask the client if he's choking and if he can speak. Next, she should administer abdominal thrusts or chest thrusts (if the client is obese or pregnant). She should continue thrusts until they're effective or until the client becomes unresponsive, at which time she should activate the emergency response team and begin to administer CPR.

CN: Physiological integrity; CNS: Physiological adaptation; CL: Application

75. A nurse is performing a cardiac assessment on a client with a suspected murmur. Identify the area where the nurse should place the stethoscope to auscultate the area referred to as *Erb's point*.

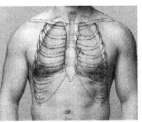

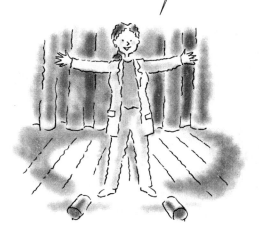

What a performance! For your first comprehensive test, that was outstanding. Congratulations!

75. Erb's point is located at the third left intercostal space, close to the sternum. Murmurs of both aortic and pulmonic origin may be heard at Erb's point.

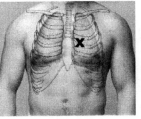

CN: Health promotion and maintenance; CNS: None; CL: Application

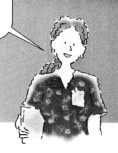

Here's another comprehensive test to help you get ready to take the NCLEX test. Good luck!

COMPREHENSIVE
Test 2

1. A newly hired GN is helping the charge nurse admit a client. The charge nurse asks the GN if she understands the facility's rules of ethical conduct. Which statement by the GN indicates the need for further teaching?
1. "I make sure that I do everything in my client's best interest."
2. "I maintain client confidentiality always."
3. "I'll support the Client's Bill of Rights."
4. "I don't discuss advance directives unless the client initiates the conversation."

2. Which diagnostic test is performed first to detect transposition of the great vessels (TGV)?
1. Blood cultures
2. Cardiac catheterization
3. Chest X-ray
4. Echocardiogram

3. Four 6-month-old children arrive at the clinic for diphtheria-pertussis-tetanus (DTaP) immunization. Which child can safely receive the immunization at this time?
1. The child with a temperature of 103° F (39.4° C)
2. The child with a runny nose
3. The child with uncontrolled epilepsy
4. The child with difficulty breathing after the last immunization

4. A nurse is giving discharge instructions to parents of a child who had a tonsillectomy. Which instruction is the most important?
1. The child should drink extra milk.
2. The child shouldn't drink from straws.
3. Orange juice should be given to provide pain control.
4. The child's mouth should be rinsed with salt water to provide pain relief.

1. 4. The law mandates that healthcare agencies ask all clients if they have an advance directive. Therefore, the nurse must address this question regardless of whether the client initiates a conversation about it. Nurses always need to act in the best interest of their clients, maintain confidentiality, and support the client's Bill of Rights.
CN: Safe, effective care environment; CNS: Management of care; CL: Analysis

2. 3. Chest X-ray would be done first to visualize congenital heart diseases such as TGV. Blood cultures won't diagnose TGV. Cardiac catheterization and an echocardiogram would be done after TGV is seen on the chest X-ray.
CN: Health promotion and maintenance; CNS: None; CL: Application

3. 2. Children with mild acute illness without fever can safely receive DTaP immunization. Children with a temperature of more than 102° F (38.9° C), uncontrolled epilepsy, or serious reactions to previous immunizations shouldn't receive DTaP immunization.
CN: Health promotion and maintenance; CNS: None; CL: Analysis

4. 2. Straws and other sharp objects inserted into the mouth could disrupt the clot at the operative site. Extra milk wouldn't promote healing and may encourage mucus production. Drinking orange juice and rinsing with salt water will irritate the tissue at the operative site.
CN: Physiological adaptation; CNS: Reduction of risk potential; CL: Application

CN: Client needs category CNS: Client needs subcategory CL: Cognitive level

5. A 2-year-old child is diagnosed with bronchiolitis caused by respiratory syncytial virus (RSV). The child's family also includes an 8-year-old child. Which statement is correct?
1. RSV isn't highly communicable in infants.
2. RSV isn't communicable to older children and adults.
3. The 2-year-old client must be admitted to the hospital for isolation.
4. The children should be separated to prevent the spread of the infection.

6. A child with asthma uses a peak expiratory flowmeter in school. The results indicate his peak flow is in the yellow zone. Which intervention by the school nurse is appropriate?
1. Follow the child's routine asthma treatment plan.
2. Monitor the child for signs and symptoms of an acute attack.
3. Call 911 and prepare for transport to the nearest emergency department.
4. Call the child's mother to take the child to the family physician immediately.

7. Parents of a child with asthma are trying to identify possible allergens in their household. Which inhaled allergen is the most common?
1. Perfume
2. Dust mites
3. Passive smoke
4. Dog or cat dander

8. A nurse is verifying orders from a physician. Which diet is correct for a child newly diagnosed with celiac disease?
1. Low-fat diet
2. No-gluten diet
3. High-protein diet
4. No-phenylalanine diet

5. 4. Toddlers easily transmit and contract RSV and so they should be separated from other children. RSV is also communicable to older children and adults, but these clients may exhibit only mild symptoms of the disorder. Hospitalization is indicated only for children who need oxygen and I.V. therapy.
CN: Safe, effective care environment; CNS: Safety and infection control; CL: Analysis

6. 2. The child should be monitored to determine if an asthma attack is imminent. The routine treatment plan may be insufficient when the peak flow is in the yellow zone (50% to 80% of personal best). This isn't an emergency situation. There's no immediate need to see the physician if the child is asymptomatic.
CN: Physiological integrity; CNS: Reduction of risk potential; CL: Application

7. 2. The household dust mite is the most commonly inhaled allergen that can cause an asthma attack. Animal dander, passive smoke, and perfume are sometimes allergens causing asthma attacks but aren't as common as dust mites.
CN: Safe, effective care environment; CNS: Safety and infection control; CL: Application

8. 2. The intestinal cells of individuals with celiac disease become inflamed when the child eats products containing gluten, such as wheat, rye, barley, or oats. The child with celiac disease needs normal amounts of fat and protein in the diet for growth and development. Omitting phenylalanine products would be appropriate for the client with phenylketonuria.
CN: Safe, effective care environment; CNS: Safety and infection control; CL: Application

9. A client is undergoing a thoracentesis at the bedside. The nurse assists the client to an upright position with a table and pillow in front of him to support his arms. Which rationale for this intervention is correct?
   1. There's easier access to the fluid from this approach.
   2. There's less chance to injure lung tissue.
   3. It prevents the formation of subcutaneous emphysema.
   4. It's less painful for the client in this position.

9. 1. The posterior approach is superior. The posterior gutter is deep and fluid tends to collect in this dependent area while the client is in an erect position. There's a risk for pneumothorax and subcutaneous emphysema formation regardless of the client's position. This procedure is done using local anesthesia, so it isn't painful.
CN: Physiological integrity; CNS: Physiological adaptation; CL: Analysis

10. Which leisure activity is recommended for a school-age child with hemophilia?
   1. Baseball
   2. Cross-country running
   3. Football
   4. Swimming

10. 4. Swimming is a noncontact sport with low risk for traumatic injury. Baseball, cross-country running, and football all involve a risk for trauma from falling, sliding, or contact.
CN: Physiological integrity; CNS: Physiological adaptation; CL: Application

11. Which assessment is important for an infant in sickle cell crisis?
   1. The infant has no bruises.
   2. The infant has normal skin turgor.
   3. The infant participates in exercise.
   4. The infant maintains bladder control.

11. 2. Normal skin turgor indicates the infant isn't severely dehydrated. Dehydration may cause sickle cell crisis or worsen a crisis. Bruising isn't associated with sickle cell crisis. Bed rest is preferable during a sickle cell crisis. Bladder control may be lost when oral or I.V. fluid intake is increased during a sickle cell crisis.
CN: Physiological integrity; CNS: Physiological adaptation; CL: Analysis

12. A client has arterial blood gases drawn. The results are as follows: pH, 7.52; Pao_2, 50 mm Hg; $Paco_2$, 28 mm Hg; HCO_3^-, 24 mEq/L. Which condition is indicated?
   1. Metabolic acidosis
   2. Metabolic alkalosis
   3. Respiratory acidosis
   4. Respiratory alkalosis

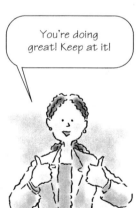

You're doing great! Keep at it!

12. 4. A pH greater than 7.45 and a $Paco_2$ less than 35 mm Hg indicate respiratory alkalosis. A pH less than 7.35 and an HCO_3^- less than 22 mEq/L indicate metabolic acidosis. A pH greater than 7.45 and an HCO_3^- greater than 24 mEq/L indicate metabolic alkalosis. A pH less than 7.35 and a $Paco_2$ greater than 45 mm Hg indicate respiratory acidosis.
CN: Physiological integrity; CNS: Reduction of risk potential; CL: Analysis

13. A client with chronic alcohol abuse is admitted to the hospital for detoxification. Later that day, his blood pressure increases and he's given lorazepam (Ativan) to prevent which complication?
   1. Stroke
   2. Seizure
   3. Fainting
   4. Anxiety reaction

13. 2. During detoxification from alcohol, changes in the client's physiologic status, especially an increase in blood pressure, may indicate a possible seizure. Clients are treated with benzodiazepines to prevent this. Stroke, fainting, and anxiety aren't the primary concerns when withdrawing from alcohol.
CN: Physiological integrity; CNS: Pharmacological and parenteral therapies; CL: Application

14. An adolescent client ingests a large number of acetaminophen (Tylenol) tablets in an attempt to commit suicide. Which laboratory result is most consistent with acetaminophen overdose?

1. Metabolic acidosis
2. Elevated liver enzyme levels
3. Increased serum creatinine level
4. Increased white blood cell (WBC) count

15. A nurse is caring for a client recently diagnosed with acute pancreatitis. Which statement indicates that a short-term goal of nursing care has been met?

1. The client denies abdominal pain.
2. The client doesn't complain of thirst.
3. The client denies pain at McBurney's point.
4. The client swallows liquids without coughing.

16. A client is to take 8 ounces of magnesium sulfate solution. The calibrations on the measuring device are in milliliters. How many milliliters should the nurse give?

1. 8 ml
2. 80 ml
3. 240 ml
4. 480 ml

17. A man stepped on a piece of sharp glass while walking barefoot. He comes to the emergency department with a deep laceration on the bottom of his foot. Which question is the most important for the nurse to ask?

1. "Was the glass dirty?"
2. "Are you immune to tetanus?"
3. "When did you have your last tetanus shot?"
4. "How many diphtheria-pertussis-tetanus (DTaP) shots did you receive as a child?"

14. 2. Elevated liver enzyme levels, which could indicate liver damage, are associated with acetaminophen overdose. Metabolic acidosis isn't associated with acetaminophen overdose. An increased serum creatinine level may indicate renal damage. An increased WBC count indicates infection.

CN: Physiological integrity; CNS: Pharmacological and parenteral therapies; CL: Application

15. 1. Pancreatitis is accompanied by acute pain from autodigestion by pancreatic enzymes. When the client denies abdominal pain, the short-term goal of pain control is met. Clients with acute pancreatitis receive I.V. fluids and may not have a sensation of thirst. Pain at McBurney's point accompanies appendicitis. Clients with acute pancreatitis receive nothing by mouth during initial therapy.

CN: Physiological integrity; CNS: Physiological adaptation; CL: Application

16. 3. To determine the amount of milliliters to give, use the following equation: One ounce = 30 ml. 8 × 30 ml = 240 ml.

CN: Physiological integrity; CNS: Pharmacological and parenteral therapies; CL: Application

17. 3. Questioning the client about the date of his last tetanus immunization is important because the booster immunization should be received every 10 years in adulthood or at the time of the injury if the last booster immunization was given more than 5 years before the injury. Whether the client noticed dirt on the glass is immaterial because all deep lacerations require a tetanus immunization or booster. A client wouldn't know his tetanus immunity status. DTaP immunizations in childhood don't give lifelong immunization to tetanus.

CN: Safe, effective care environment; CNS: Safety and infection control; CL: Application

18. A postmenopausal client asks a nurse how to prevent osteoporosis. Which response is best?
1. "Take a multivitamin daily."
2. "After menopause, there's no way to prevent osteoporosis."
3. "Drink two glasses of milk each day and swim three times a week."
4. "Do weight-bearing exercises regularly."

18. 4. Weight-bearing exercises are recommended for the prevention of osteoporosis. Telling the client that there's no way to prevent osteoporosis would be an incorrect statement. A multivitamin doesn't provide adequate calcium for a post-menopausal woman, and calcium alone won't prevent osteoporosis. Two glasses of milk per day don't provide the daily requirements for adult women, and swimming isn't a weight-bearing exercise.
CN: Health promotion and maintenance; CNS: None; CL: Application

19. A client diagnosed with cardiomyopathy saw a posting on the Internet describing research about a new herbal treatment for the disorder. When the client asks about this research, which response is most appropriate?
1. "Herbs are often used to treat cardiomyopathy."
2. "Cardiomyopathy can be treated only by heart surgery."
3. "The Internet is a reliable source of research, so try this treatment."
4. "Research found on the Internet should be verified with a physician."

19. 4. Although the Internet contains some valid medical research, there's no control over the validity of information posted on it. The research should be discussed with a physician who has access to medical research and can verify the accuracy of the information. Herbs aren't standard treatment for cardiomyopathy. Cardiomyopathy is treatable with drugs or surgery.
CN: Safe, effective care environment; CNS: Management of care; CL: Application

20. A young adult client received her first chemotherapy treatment for breast cancer. Which statement, if made by the client, requires further exploration by the nurse?
1. "I'm thinking about joining a dance club."
2. "I don't think I'm going to work tomorrow."
3. "I don't care about the side effects of drugs."
4. "I want to return to school for a college degree."

20. 3. Adverse effects of chemotherapy may occur after treatment and should be discussed with the client because some can be treated, controlled, or prevented. The nurse needs to explore what the client means by this statement. Joining social clubs is typical behavior for a young adult. The client may feel poorly after chemotherapy and may want to take time off from work until feeling better. Returning to school is also typical of a young adult.
CN: Health promotion and maintenance; CNS: None; CL: Analysis

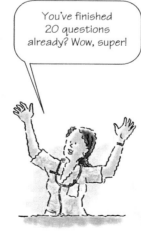

You've finished 20 questions already? Wow, super!

21. A male client has been diagnosed with panhypopituitarism. Which hormone will be given to the client orally?
1. Estrogen
2. Levothyroxine (Synthroid)
3. Serotonin
4. Testosterone

21. 2. Thyroid hormone release depends on the release of thyroid-stimulating hormone (TSH) by the anterior pituitary. TSH is absent from the pituitary when panhypopituitarism exists, so levothyroxine should be given orally. Estrogen isn't indicated for a male client. Serotonin release isn't controlled by the pituitary gland. Testosterone is given by injection or topically by patch.
CN: Physiological integrity; CNS: Pharmacological and parenteral therapies; CL: Application

CN: Client needs category   CNS: Client needs subcategory   CL: Cognitive level

22. Which nursing intervention is appropriate for an adult client with chronic renal failure?
1. Weigh the client daily before breakfast.
2. Offer foods high in calcium and phosphorous.
3. Serve the client large meals and a bedtime snack.
4. Encourage the client to drink large amounts of fluids.

23. A physician prescribes acetaminophen (Tylenol) gr X (10 grains) as necessary every 4 hours for pain for a client in a long-term care facility. How many milligrams of acetaminophen should the nurse give? Record your answer using a whole number:

_____ mg.

24. Which assessment finding indicates an increased risk for skin cancer?
1. A deep sunburn
2. A dark mole on the client's back
3. An irregular scar on the client's abdomen
4. White irregular patches on the client's arm

25. Which behavior is consistent with the diagnosis of conduct disorder in a child?
1. Enuresis
2. Suicidal ideation
3. Cruelty to animals
4. Fear of going to school

26. Which symptom is associated with a genital chlamydia infection?
1. Genital warts
2. No symptoms
3. Purulent discharge
4. Fluid-filled blisters

22. 1. Daily weights are obtained to monitor fluid retention. Calcium intake is encouraged, but clients with chronic renal failure have difficulty excreting phosphorous. Therefore, phosphorous must be restricted. To improve food intake, meals and snacks should be given in small portions. Fluids should be restricted for the client with chronic renal failure.
CN: Physiological integrity; CNS: Physiological adaptation; CL: Application

23. 650 mg. To determine the amount of milligrams to give, use the following equation:

One grain = 65 mg

$$\frac{1\ gr}{65\ mg} \times \frac{10\ gr}{x\ mg}$$

$$X = 65 \times 10$$
$$X = 650\ mg$$

CN: Physiological integrity; CNS: Pharmacological and parenteral therapies; CL: Application

24. 1. A deep sunburn is a risk factor for skin cancer. A dark mole or an irregular scar are benign findings. White irregular patches are abnormal but aren't a risk factor for skin cancer.
CN: Health promotion and maintenance; CNS: None; CL: Application

25. 3. Cruelty to animals is a symptom of conduct disorder. Enuresis and suicidal ideation aren't usually associated with conduct disorder. Fear of going to school is school phobia.
CN: Psychosocial integrity; CNS: None; CL: Application

26. 3. Purulent discharge from the cervix, urethra, or Bartholin's gland is associated with several sexually transmitted diseases, including chlamydia. Genital warts are a sign of human papillomavirus. Although some women with genital chlamydia infection are asymptomatic, this isn't the usual course of this condition. Fluid-filled blisters are a sign of herpes infection.
CN: Health promotion and maintenance; CNS: None; CL: Application

27. Which outcome is appropriate for a client with a diagnosis of depression and attempted suicide?
1. The client will never feel suicidal again.
2. The client will find a group home to live in.
3. The client will remain hospitalized for at least 6 months.
4. The client will verbalize an absence of suicidal ideation, plan, and intent.

28. The nurse is reviewing the proper technique in obtaining a urine specimen from an indwelling urinary catheter. When collecting the urine, which would be the most appropriate technique to use?
1. Collect urine from the drainage collection bag.
2. Disconnect the catheter from the drainage tubing to collect urine.
3. Remove the indwelling catheter and insert a sterile straight catheter to collect urine.
4. Insert a sterile needle with syringe through a tubing drainage port cleaned with alcohol to collect the specimen.

29. A registered nurse (RN) is supervising the care of a licensed practical nurse (LPN). The LPN is caring for a client diagnosed with a terminal illness. Which statement by the LPN should be corrected by the RN?
1. "Some clients write a living will indicating their end-of-life preferences."
2. "The law says you have to write a new living will each time you go to the hospital."
3. "You could designate another person to make end-of-life decisions when you can't make them yourself."
4. "Some people choose to tell their physician they don't want to have cardiopulmonary resuscitation."

30. An elderly client's husband tells a nurse he's concerned because his wife insists on talking about events that happened to her years in the past. The nurse assesses the client and finds her alert, oriented, and answering questions appropriately. Which statement made to the husband is correct?
1. "Your wife is reviewing her life."
2. "A spiritual advisor should be notified."
3. "Your wife should be discouraged from talking about the past."
4. "Your wife is regressing to a more comfortable time in the past."

27. 4. An appropriate outcome is that the client will verbalize that he no longer feels suicidal. It's unrealistic to ask that he never feels suicidal again. There's no reason for a group home or 6 months of hospitalization.
CN: Psychosocial integrity; CNS: None; CL: Application

28. 4. Wearing clean gloves, cleaning the port with alcohol, and then obtaining the specimen with a sterile needle and syringe ensures that the specimen and closed drainage system won't be contaminated. A urine specimen must be new urine, and the urine in the drainage collection bag could be several hours' old and growing bacteria. The urinary drainage system must be kept closed to prevent microorganisms from entering. It isn't necessary to remove an indwelling catheter to obtain a sterile urine specimen, unless the physician requests that the system be changed.
CN: Safe, effective care environment; CNS: Safety and infection control; CL: Application

29. 2. One living will is sufficient for all hospitalizations unless the client wishes to make changes. A living will explains a person's end-of-life preferences. A durable power of attorney for health care can be written to designate who will make health care decisions for the client in the event the client can't make decisions for himself. The "No-Code" or "Do-Not-Resuscitate" status is discussed with the physician, who then enters this in the client's chart.
CN: Safe, effective care environment; CNS: Management of care; CL: Analysis

30. 1. Life review or reminiscing is characteristic of elderly people and the dying. A spiritual advisor might comfort the client but isn't necessary for a life review. Discouraging the client from talking would block communication. Regression occurs when a client returns to behaviors typical of another developmental stage.
CN: Health promotion and maintenance; CNS: None; CL: Application

CN: Client needs category   CNS: Client needs subcategory   CL: Cognitive level

31. A client with a new colostomy asks a nurse how to avoid leakage from the ostomy bag. Which instruction is correct?
1. Limit fluid intake.
2. Eat more fruits and vegetables.
3. Empty the bag when it's about half full.
4. Tape the end of the bag to the surrounding skin.

32. A nurse must obtain the blood pressure of a client in airborne isolation. Which method is best to prevent transmission of infection to other clients by the equipment?
1. Dispose of the equipment after each use.
2. Wear gloves while handling the equipment.
3. Use the equipment only with other clients in airborne isolation.
4. Leave the equipment in the room for use only with that client.

33. To prevent circulatory impairment in an arm when applying an elastic bandage, which method is best?
1. Wrap the bandage around the arm loosely.
2. Apply the bandage while stretching it slightly.
3. Apply heavy pressure with each turn of the bandage.
4. Start applying the bandage at the upper arm and work toward the lower arm.

34. The physician's order reads: 2 grams of cephalexin (Keflex) P.O. daily in equally divided doses of 500 mg each. The nurse would administer this medication at which frequency?
1. 3 times per day
2. 4 times per day
3. 6 times per day
4. 8 times per day

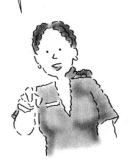

I'm so proud of you. Keep up the good work!

31. 3. Emptying the bag when partially full will prevent the bag from becoming heavy and detaching from the skin or skin barrier. Limiting fluids may cause constipation but won't prevent leakage. Increasing fruits and vegetables in the diet will help prevent constipation, not leakage. Taping the bag to the skin will secure the bag to the skin but won't prevent leakage.
CN: Physiological integrity; CNS: Basic care and comfort; CL: Application

32. 4. Leaving equipment in the room is appropriate to avoid organism transmission by inanimate objects. Disposing of equipment after each use prevents the transmission of organisms but isn't cost-effective. Wearing gloves protects the nurse, not other clients. Using equipment for other clients spreads infectious organisms among clients.
CN: Safe, effective care environment; CNS: Safety and infection control; CL: Application

33. 2. Stretching the bandage slightly maintains uniform tension on the bandage. Wrapping the bandage loosely wouldn't secure the bandage on the arm. Using heavy pressure would cause circulatory impairment. Beginning the wrapping at the upper arm would cause uneven application of the bandage. For example, elastic stockings are applied distal to proximal to promote venous return.
CN: Physiological integrity; CNS: Reduction of risk potential; CL: Application

34. 2. 2 grams is equivalent to 2,000 mg (1 gm = 1,000 mg). To give equally divided doses of 500 mg, divide the desired dose of 500 mg into the total daily dose of 2,000 mg. This gives an answer of 4, which is the number of times this dose of medication will be administered per day. This means giving 500 mg every 6 hours, for a total of 4 times per day.
CN: Physiological integrity; CNS: Pharmacological and parenteral therapies; CL: Analysis

35. A client complains of an inability to sleep while on the medical unit. Which intervention should be performed first?
1. Offer a sedative routinely at bedtime.
2. Give the client a backrub before bedtime.
3. Question the client about sleeping habits.
4. Move the client to a bed farthest from the nurses' station.

36. In order to assess the function of a client's optic nerve, the nurse would be required to use which equipment?
1. Finger, to test the cardinal fields
2. Flashlight, to test corneal reflexes
3. Snellen's chart, to test visual acuity
4. Piece of cotton, to test corneal sensitivity

37. A nurse is caring for a client following surgery in the post-anesthesia care unit. The nurse observes that the client is gagging on his airway and about to vomit. In which position would the nurse place the client?
1. Prone
2. Trendelenburg
3. Supine
4. Recovery

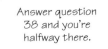

Answer question 38 and you're halfway there.

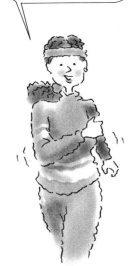

38. Which intervention is best to prevent bladder infections for a client with an indwelling urinary catheter?
1. Limit fluid intake.
2. Encourage showers rather than tub baths.
3. Open the drainage system to obtain a urine specimen.
4. Irrigate the catheter twice daily with sterile saline solution.

39. A nurse wants to use a waist restraint for a client who wanders at night. Which factor or intervention should be considered before applying the restraint?
1. The nurse's convenience
2. The client's reason for getting out of bed
3. A sleeping medication ordered as needed at bedtime
4. The lack of nursing assistants on the night shift

35. 3. Interviewing the client about sleeping habits may give more information about the causes of the inability to sleep. Sedatives should be given as a last option. A backrub may promote sleep but may not address this client's problem. Moving the client may not address the client's specific problem.
CN: Physiological integrity; CNS: Basic care and comfort; CL: Application

36. 3. The Snellen's chart is used to test the function of the optic nerve. Testing the cardinal fields assesses the oculomotor, trochlear, and abducens nerves. Corneal light reflex reflects the function of the oculomotor nerve. Corneal sensitivity is controlled by the trigeminal and facial nerves.
CN: Health promotion and maintenance; CNS: None; CL: Application

37. 4. Unless contraindicated, the recovery position, or right- or left-side lying position, should be used. This position is commonly called the recovery position because it is used to prevent aspiration of secretions or vomitus during the postoperative phase. The prone position is face down and not appropriate. Trendelenburg position is used for shock and supine position places the client flat on their back making aspiration possible.
CN: Physiological integrity; CNS: Reduction of risk potential; CL: Application

38. 2. A shower would prevent bacteria in the bath water from sustaining contact with the urinary meatus and the catheter, while a tub bath may allow easier transit of bacteria into the urinary tract. Increased—not limited—fluid intake is recommended for a client with an indwelling urinary catheter. Opening the drainage system would provide a pathway for the entry of bacteria. Catheter irrigation is performed only with an order from the physician to keep the catheter patent.
CN: Physiological integrity; CNS: Reduction of risk potential; CL: Comprehension

39. 2. The nurse should question the client's reason for getting out of bed because the client may be looking for a bathroom. Lack of adequate staffing and convenience aren't reasons for applying restraints. Sleeping medications are chemical restraints that should be used only if the client is unable to go to sleep and stay asleep.
CN: Safe, effective care environment; CNS: Safety and infection control; CL: Application

CN: Client needs category   CNS: Client needs subcategory   CL: Cognitive level

40. Six months after the death of her infant son, a client is suspected of dysfunctional grieving. Which assessment would the nurse expect to find in this client?
1. She goes to the infant's grave weekly.
2. She cries when talking about the loss.
3. She's overactive without a sense of loss.
4. She states the infant will always be part of the family.

41. A nurse notices a client has been crying. Which response is most therapeutic?
1. None; this is a private matter.
2. "You seem sad, would you like to talk?"
3. "Why are you crying and upsetting yourself?"
4. "It's hard being in the hospital, but you must keep your chin up."

42. A nurse gives the wrong medication to a client. Another nurse employed by the hospital as a risk manager will expect to receive which communication?
1. Incident report
2. Oral report from the nurse
3. Copy of the medication Kardex
4. Order change signed by the physician

43. A student nurse wants to know what charge can result from performing a procedure on a client in the absence of informed consent. Which response by the nurse is accurate?
1. Fraud
2. Harassment
3. Assault and battery
4. Breach of confidentiality

44. A surgical client newly diagnosed with cancer tells a nurse she knows the laboratory made a mistake about her diagnosis. Which reaction is this client most likely experiencing?
1. Denial
2. Intellectualization
3. Regression
4. Repression

40. 3. One of the signs of dysfunctional grieving is overactivity without a sense of loss. Including the infant as a part of the family, going to the grave, and crying are all normal responses.
CN: Psychosocial integrity; CNS: None; CL: Application

41. 2. Therapeutic communication is a primary tool of nursing. The nurse must recognize the client's nonverbal behaviors indicate a need to talk. Asking "why" is often interpreted as an accusation. Ignoring the client's nonverbal cues or giving opinions and advice are barriers to communication.
CN: Psychosocial integrity; CNS: None; CL: Application

42. 1. Incident reports are tools used by risk managers when a client might be harmed. They're used to determine how future problems can be avoided. An oral report won't serve as legal documentation. A copy of the medication Kardex wouldn't be sent with the incident report to the risk manager. A physician won't change an order to cover the nurse's mistake.
CN: Safe, effective care environment; CNS: Management of care; CL: Application

43. 3. Performing a procedure on a client without informed consent can be grounds for charges of assault and battery. Fraud is to cheat, harassment means to annoy or disturb, and breach of confidentiality refers to conveying information about the client.
CN: Safe, effective care environment; CNS: Management of care; CL: Application

44. 1. Cancer clients often deny this diagnosis when first made. Such a response may benefit the client in that it allows energy for surgical healing. Repression describes not remembering being diagnosed, regression describes childlike behavior, and intellectualization describes speaking of the disease as if reading a textbook.
CN: Psychosocial integrity; CNS: None; CL: Application

45. An unmarried client delivers a premature neonate. Which intervention is included in her treatment plan?
1. An early postpartum physician visit
2. Referral to the health department
3. Request for a social service visit in the hospital
4. Request for a home health visit the day after discharge

46. Which statement made by a client about her neonate indicates the need for further teaching?
1. "I'll trim the baby's nails when he's sleeping."
2. "I'll remember to place the baby on his back when he sleeps."
3. "Our infant car seat must be placed in the back seat of the car."
4. "The first thing I'm going to do when we get home is give the baby a tub bath."

47. A client in labor is receiving oxytocin (Pitocin) to augment her labor. A nurse notes a change in her contraction pattern. The fetal heart monitor indicates that her contractions are lasting 2 minutes, with a notable rise in the baseline. Based on this finding, which action is the priority?
1. Notify the physician.
2. Give oxygen through a mask.
3. Turn oxytocin to the lowest level.
4. Turn the client on her left side.

48. A client who just gave birth is concerned about her neonate's Apgar scores of 7 and 8. She says she's been told scores lower than 9 are associated with learning difficulties in later life. Which response is best?
1. "You shouldn't worry so much, your infant is perfectly fine."
2. "You should ask about placing the infant in a follow-up diagnostic program."
3. "You're right in being concerned, but there are good special education programs available."
4. "Apgar scores are used to indicate a need for resuscitation at birth. Scores of 7 and above indicate no problem."

45. 3. Due to the client's marital status and premature condition of the neonate, a social service visit is appropriate. The social service visit will determine if there's a need for a referral to the health department. The mother has no physical indications for an early postpartum visit or need for an early home visit.
CN: Safe, effective care environment; CNS: Management of care; CL: Analysis

46. 4. Neonates shouldn't be placed in a tub bath until after the cord falls off and is completely healed to prevent infection. It's correct to cut his nails while he sleeps, place a neonate on his back, and place the car seat in the back.
CN: Safe, effective care environment; CNS: Safety and infection control; CL: Analysis

47. 3. The first action must be to lower the oxytocin, to prevent fetal hypoxia or possible rupture of the uterus. The client would then be placed on her left side, given oxygen to prevent fetal hypoxia, and the physician would be notified.
CN: Safe, effective care environment; CNS: Management of care; CL: Analysis

48. 4. Apgar scores don't indicate future learning difficulties; they're for rapid assessment of the need for resuscitation. It's inappropriate to just tell a client not to worry. An Apgar score of 7 and 8 is normal and doesn't indicate a need for intervention.
CN: Health promotion and maintenance; CNS: None; CL: Application

CN: Client needs category   CNS: Client needs subcategory   CL: Cognitive level

49. After delivering a neonate with a cleft palate and cleft lip, a client has minimal contact with her neonate. She asks the nurse to do most of the neonate's care. Which nursing diagnosis is appropriate?
1. *Anxiety related to fear of harming the neonate*
2. *Deficient knowledge related to neonate's potential*
3. *Risk for impaired parenting related to birth defect*
4. *Ineffective coping related to birth defect*

50. A breast-feeding client asks how she can do breast self-examination (BSE) while nursing. Which response would be the most accurate?
1. "You should do BSE after the infant has emptied the breast."
2. "You don't have to do BSE until after you stop breast-feeding."
3. "You should continue to do BSE the way you did before becoming pregnant."
4. "Your physician will examine your breasts until after you stop breast-feeding."

51. A prenatal client says she can't believe she has such mixed feelings about being pregnant. She tried for 10 years to become pregnant and now she feels guilty for her conflicting reactions. Which response is best?
1. "You need to talk to your midwife about these feelings."
2. "You're experiencing the normal ambivalence pregnant mothers feel."
3. "These feelings are expected only in women who have had difficulty becoming pregnant."
4. "Let's make an appointment with a counselor."

52. A maternity client says her husband is behaving in strange ways since she became pregnant. He's having morning sickness, has put on weight, complains of intestinal pains, and is acting like he's pregnant. Which term describes this reaction?
1. Extreme anxiety
2. Normal couvade
3. Signs of reaction formation
4. Abnormal, needing counseling

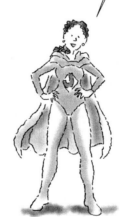

You've now completed 50 questions and are two-thirds finished. Super!

49. 3. Neonates born with birth defects are at risk for impaired parenting. The parents must work through issues of not producing the perfect child and guilt associated with this. There's nothing in the question that indicates the client felt anxious about caring for the neonate or had ineffective coping problems or a knowledge deficit.
CN: Safe, effective care environment; CNS: Management of care; CL: Application

50. 1. During breast-feeding, the client should examine each breast after the neonate has emptied the breast. Women must continue to examine their breasts, even if they're lactating. Contrary to how it's performed before pregnancy, BSE should be done on the same day of the month until the menstrual cycle returns. Breast examination shouldn't be done solely by the physician.
CN: Health promotion and maintenance; CNS: None; CL: Application

51. 2. Conflicting, ambivalent feelings regarding pregnancy are normal for all pregnant women. These feelings don't call for counseling or other professional interventions. Ambivalence is felt by most pregnant women, not only mothers who had difficulty becoming pregnant.
CN: Psychosocial integrity; CNS: None; CL: Application

52. 2. The father's adjustment may include behaviors referred to as couvade. Historically, there have been different cultural couvades. Today, the term is associated with the father developing pregnancy-like symptoms. Because the behavior is normal and isn't reaction formation or anxiety, there's no need for counseling.
CN: Psychosocial integrity; CNS: None; CL: Analysis

53. Three days after discharge, a client bottle-feeding her neonate calls the postpartum floor, asking what she can do for breast engorgement. Which instruction is correct?
1. Put a tight binder around her breasts.
2. Get under a warm shower and let the water flow on her breasts.
3. Stop drinking milk because it contributes to breast engorgement.
4. Contact her physician; she shouldn't be engorged at this late date.

54. A pregnant client complains of leg cramps that wake her from sleep. Which instruction is correct?
1. Dorsiflex the foot.
2. Elevate the legs at night.
3. Point the toes until the cramp releases.
4. Drink more than 1 quart of milk a day.

55. A client is being treated for premature labor with ritodrine (Yutopar). After receiving this medication for 12 hours, her blood pressure is slightly elevated, her chest is clear, and her pulse is 120 beats/minute. She complains of a little nausea, and the fetal heart rate is 145 beats/minute. Which intervention is correct?
1. Continue routine monitoring.
2. Contact the physician immediately.
3. Turn the client on her left side and give oxygen.
4. Increase the flow rate of the I.V. and give oxygen.

56. At 6 cm of dilation, the client in labor receives a lumbar epidural for pain control. Which nursing diagnosis is possible?
1. Risk for injury related to rapid delivery
2. Acute pain related to wearing off of anesthesia
3. Hyperthermia related to effects of anesthesia
4. Ineffective peripheral tissue perfusion related to effects of anesthesia

53. 1. A tight binder is recommended for the client bottle-feeding her neonate to reduce engorgement. A warm shower will stimulate milk production. It's normal to become engorged during the first few days after delivery, and drinking milk isn't the cause.
CN: Physiological integrity; CNS: Basic care and comfort; CL: Application

54. 1. Dorsiflexion of the foot is the recommended intervention to relieve a leg cramp during pregnancy. Elevating the legs isn't a usual treatment. Drinking more than 1 quart of milk and pointing the toes are associated with causing leg cramps.
CN: Physiological integrity; CNS: Basic care and comfort; CL: Application

55. 1. These findings are normal adverse effects to the medication and don't call for interventions at this time except to continue routine monitoring. Contacting the physician, placing the client on her left side, changing the I.V. flow rate, and giving oxygen are all interventions for abnormal assessment findings.
CN: Physiological integrity; CNS: Pharmacological and parental therapies; CL: Analysis

56. 4. A disadvantage of a lumbar epidural is the risk for hypotension, which can lead to ineffective tissue perfusion. Epidurals are associated with a longer labor and hypothermia. There's no pain involved with the anesthesia wearing off.
CN: Safe, effective care environment; CNS: Management of care; CL: Application

CN: Client needs category CNS: Client needs subcategory CL: Cognitive level

57. When assessing a client who just delivered a neonate, a nurse finds the following: blood pressure, 110/70 mm Hg; pulse, 60 beats/minute; respirations, 16 breaths/minute; lochia, moderate rubra; fundus, above the umbilicus to the right; and negative Homans' sign. Which intervention is correct?
   1. Nothing; all findings are normal.
   2. Have the client void and recheck the fundus.
   3. Turn the client on her left side to decrease the blood pressure.
   4. Rub the fundus to decrease lochia flow and prevent hemorrhage.

58. A client with diabetes delivers a 9-lb, 6-oz neonate. The neonate is assessed for which condition?
   1. Hyperglycemia
   2. Hypoglycemia
   3. Hyperthermia
   4. Hypothermia

59. A prenatal client, age 13, asks about getting fat while she's pregnant. A nurse tells her she needs to gain enough weight to be in the upper portions of her recommended weight due to her age to prevent which condition?
   1. Delivery of a premature neonate
   2. A difficult delivery
   3. Delivery of a low birth-weight neonate
   4. Gestational hypertension

60. A mother of a neonate receiving phototherapy asks why her child has developed loose stools. Which response by the nurse would be accurate?
   1. They're abnormal and may indicate an infection.
   2. They're associated with an adverse reaction to formula.
   3. They're common when receiving phototherapy treatments.
   4. They're abnormal and phototherapy should be discontinued.

57. 2. A fundus up and to the right indicates a full bladder. The client should empty her bladder and be reassessed. Lochia flow and blood pressure are normal.
CN: Physiological integrity; CNS: Reduction of risk potential; CL: Analysis

58. 2. Neonates of mothers with diabetes and large neonates are at risk for hypoglycemia related to increased production of insulin by the neonate in utero. Hyperglycemia, hypothermia, and hyperthermia aren't primary concerns.
CN: Physiological integrity; CNS: Reduction of risk potential; CL: Application

59. 3. Adolescent girls, especially those younger than age 15, are at higher risk for delivering low birth-weight neonates unless they gain adequate weight during pregnancy. Gaining weight isn't associated with having an easier delivery, risk for gestational hypertension, or risk of delivering a premature neonate.
CN: Physiological integrity; CNS: Reduction of risk potential; CL: Application

60. 3. While receiving phototherapy, a breakdown of bilirubin often results in loose stools. The neonate must be monitored for diarrhea and dehydration when under the lights. The loose stools wouldn't be considered related to infection or formula at this time.
CN: Physiological integrity; CNS: Physiological adaptation; CL: Application

61. A client at 36 weeks' gestation chokes on her food while eating at a restaurant. Which statement is correct about performing the Heimlich maneuver on a pregnant client?
1. Chest thrusts are used when the client is pregnant.
2. Only back thrusts are used when the client is pregnant.
3. The Heimlich maneuver is performed the same as when not pregnant.
4. The Heimlich maneuver can't be performed on a pregnant client.

62. A nurse is reviewing principles of good body mechanics with a student nurse. Which of the following techniques should be emphasized?
1. Bending from the waist
2. Pulling rather than pushing
3. Stretching to reach an object
4. Using large muscles in the legs for leverage

63. A client with a substance abuse problem is being discharged from the state mental hospital. The client's discharge plans should include which intervention?
1. Referral to Al-Anon
2. Weekly urine testing for drug use
3. Day hospital treatment for 6 months
4. Participation in a support group like Alcoholics Anonymous (AA)

64. A community mental health nurse visits a client diagnosed with paranoid schizophrenia. When she arrives at his house, he calls her Satan, shouts at her, and tells her to back away. Which intervention should be performed first?
1. Use his phone and call the police.
2. Remain safe by leaving the house.
3. Talk to him in a calm voice to reduce his agitation.
4. Remind him who she is and that he has nothing to fear.

61. 1. During pregnancy, chest thrusts are used instead of abdominal thrusts. Abdominal thrusts compress the abdomen, which would harm the fetus. Because of this, the Heimlich is adjusted for the pregnant woman. A fist is made with one hand, placing thumb side against the center of the breastbone. The fist is grabbed with the other hand and thrust inward. Avoid the lower tip of the breastbone. Back thrusts aren't done as they may result in dislodgment of the obstruction, further obstructing the airway.
CN: Physiological integrity; CNS: Reduction of risk potential; CL: Application

62. 4. Keeping one's back straight and using the large muscles in the legs will help avoid back injury, as the muscles in one's back are relatively small compared with the larger muscles of the thighs. Bending from the waist can cause stress on the back muscles, causing a potential injury. Pulling isn't the best option and may cause straining. When feasible, one should push an object rather than pull it. Stretching to reach an object increases the risk of injury.
CN: Safe, effective care environment; CNS: Safety and infection control; CL: Application

63. 4. AA is a major support group for alcoholics after treatment. Membership in AA is associated with relapse prevention. Al-Anon is a support group for the family of the abuser of alcohol. Weekly urine testing or day hospital treatment isn't usual.
CN: Safe, effective care environment; CNS: Management of care; CL: Application

64. 2. Safety is the first priority during any home visit, so the nurse should leave. Attempting to talk with the client, reminding him who she is, or using the phone places the nurse at risk for harm. After the nurse has ensured her safety, arrangements should be made to provide help for the client.
CN: Safe, effective care environment; CNS: Safety and infection control; CL: Analysis

CN: Client needs category   CNS: Client needs subcategory   CL: Cognitive level

65. A client is scheduled to retire in the next month. He phones his nurse therapist and says he can't cope; his whole world is falling apart. The therapist recognizes this reaction as which condition?
1. Panic reaction
2. Situational crisis
3. Normal separation anxiety
4. Maturational crisis

66. A client with a phobic condition is being treated with behavior modification therapy. Which treatment is expected?
1. Dream analysis
2. Free association
3. Systematic desensitization
4. Electroconvulsive therapy (ECT)

67. A severely depressed client rarely leaves his chair. To prevent physiologic complications associated with psychomotor retardation, which goal is appropriate?
1. Restrict coffee intake.
2. Increase calcium intake.
3. Rest in bed three times per day.
4. Empty the bladder on a schedule.

68. During the termination phase of a therapeutic nurse-client relationship, which intervention is avoided?
1. Refer the client to support groups.
2. Address new issues with the client.
3. Review what has been accomplished during this relationship.
4. Have the client express sadness that the relationship is ending.

69. The behavior of a client with borderline personality disorder causes a nurse to feel angry toward the client. Which response, if made by the nurse, is the most therapeutic?
1. Ignore the client's irritating behavior.
2. Restrict the client to her room until supper.
3. Report her feelings to the client's physician.
4. Tell the client how her behavior makes the nurse feel.

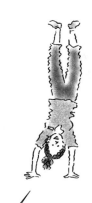

Only 10 more to go! Oh my, I just can't wait!

65. 4. A maturational (developmental) crisis is one that occurs at a predictable milestone during a life span; birth, marriage, and retirement are examples. A panic reaction would also involve physical symptoms. Situational crisis is caused by events such as an earthquake. Separation anxiety is a childhood disorder.
CN: Health promotion and maintenance; CNS: None; CL: Analysis

66. 3. Systematic desensitization is a behavior therapy used in the treatment of phobias. Dream analysis and free association are techniques used in psychoanalytic therapy. ECT is used with depression.
CN: Psychosocial integrity; CNS: None; CL: Comprehension

67. 4. To prevent bladder infections associated with stasis of urine, the client should be encouraged to routinely empty his bladder. Neither calcium nor coffee intake are directly related to the psychological effects associated with this condition. Resting in bed is another form of psychomotor retardation.
CN: Health promotion and maintenance; CNS: None; CL: Application

68. 2. During the termination phase, new issues shouldn't be explored. It's appropriate to refer the client to support groups. To review what has been accomplished is a goal of this phase. Sadness is a normal response.
CN: Psychosocial integrity; CNS: None; CL: Application

69. 4. A nursing intervention used with personality disorders is to help the client recognize how her behavior affects others. Restricting the client to her room, ignoring the client, and reporting feelings to the physician aren't appropriate interventions at this time.
CN: Psychosocial integrity; CNS: None; CL: Application

70. During a manic state, a client paced around the dayroom for 3 days. He talked to the furniture, proclaimed he was a king, and refused to partake in unit activities. Which nursing diagnosis has priority?
1. Impaired verbal communication related to hyperactivity
2. Risk for self-directed violence related to manic state
3. Imbalanced nutrition: Less than body requirements related to hyperactivity
4. Ineffective coping related to manic state

71. A client with a panic disorder is having difficulty falling asleep. Which nursing intervention should be performed first?
1. Call the client's psychotherapist.
2. Teach the client progressive relaxation.
3. Allow the client to stay up and watch television.
4. Obtain an order for a sleeping medication as needed.

72. After electroconvulsive therapy (ECT) which nursing intervention is correct?
1. Assessing the client's vital signs
2. Letting the client sleep undisturbed
3. Allowing the family to visit immediately
4. Restraining the client until completely awake

73. A client diagnosed with bipolar disease is receiving a maintenance dosage of lithium carbonate (Lithobid). His wife calls the community mental health nurse to report that her husband is hyperactive and hyperverbal. Which intervention is appropriate?
1. Mental status examination
2. Measurement of lithium blood levels
3. Evaluation at the local emergency department (ED)
4. Admission to the hospital for observation

70. 3. During a manic state, clients are at risk for malnutrition due to not taking in enough calories for the energy they're expending. The client is not displaying impaired verbal communication. This client isn't showing self-directed violent behavior. Individual coping issues aren't the primary concern at this time.
CN: Safe, effective care environment; CNS: Management of care; CL: Application

71. 2. Relaxation techniques work very well with a client showing anxiety. If this doesn't work, then contacting the psychotherapist, diversionary activities, and pharmacological interventions would be in order.
CN: Psychological integrity; CNS: None; CL: Application

72. 1. Vital signs are monitored carefully for approximately 1 hour after ECT or until the client is stable. The client shouldn't be restrained or left alone. Visitors should be allowed when the client is awake and ready.
CN: Physiological integrity; CNS: Reduction of risk potential; CL: Application

73. 2. Increased activity might indicate a need for an increased dose of lithium or that the client isn't taking his medications; blood levels will determine this. The client doesn't need to have a mental status examination, go to the ED, or be admitted to the hospital at this time.
CN: Physiological integrity; CNS: Pharmacological and parenteral therapies; CL: Analysis

74. A nurse is caring for a client with emphysema. Which nursing interventions are appropriate? Select all that apply:

1. Reduce fluid intake to less than 2,500 ml/day.
2. Teach diaphragmatic, pursed-lip breathing.
3. Administer low-flow oxygen.
4. Keep the client in a supine position as much as possible.
5. Encourage alternating activity with rest periods.
6. Teach the use of postural drainage and chest physiotherapy.

74. 2, 3, 5, 6. Diaphragmatic, pursed-lip breathing strengthens respiratory muscles and enhances oxygenation in clients with emphysema. Low-flow oxygen should be administered because a client with emphysema has chronic hypercapnia and a hypoxic respiratory drive. Alternating activity with rest allows the client to perform activities without excessive distress. If the client has copious secretions and has difficulty mobilizing them, the nurse should teach him and his family members how to perform postural drainage and chest physiotherapy. Fluid intake should be increased to 3,000 ml/day, if not contraindicated, to liquefy secretions and facilitate their removal. The client should be placed in high-Fowler's position to improve ventilation.

CN: Physiological integrity; CNS: Basic care and comfort; CL: Application

75. A nurse is assessing the abdomen of a client who was admitted to the emergency department with suspected appendicitis. Identify the area of the abdomen that the nurse should palpate last.

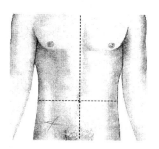

75. An acute attack of appendicitis localizes as pain and tenderness in the lower right quadrant, midway between the umbilicus and the crest of the ilium. This area should be palpated last in order to determine if pain is also present in other areas of the abdomen.

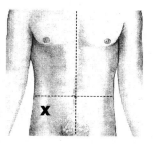

CN: Health promotion and maintenance; CNS: None; CL: Application

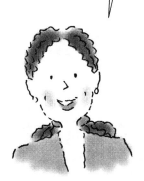

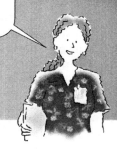

COMPREHENSIVE
Test 3

1. A client in the postoperative phase of abdominal surgery is to advance his diet as tolerated. The client has tolerated ice chips and a clear liquid diet. Which diet would the nurse expect the client to be given when he advances from this diet?
1. Fluid restricted
2. Full liquids
3. General
4. Soft

2. The following information is recorded on an intake and output record: milk, 180 ml; orange juice, 60 ml; 1 serving scrambled eggs; 1 slice toast; 1 can Ensure oral nutritional supplement, 240 ml; I.V. dextrose 5% in water at 100 ml/hour; 50 ml water after twice daily medications. Medications are given at 9:00 a.m. and 9:00 p.m. What is the client's total intake for the 7 a.m. to 3 p.m. shift?
1. 1,000 ml
2. 1,250 ml
3. 1,330 ml
4. 1,380 ml

3. A pediatrician writes an order for digoxin (Lanoxin), 2.5 mg, for a neonate. A nurse questions the order with the pharmacist and physician taking the call. Which legal standard is most relevant?
1. American Medical Association
2. American Nurses Association (ANA)
3. American Pharmaceutical Association
4. Nurse Practice Act

1. 2. Clear liquid diets are nutritionally inadequate but minimally irritating to the stomach. Clients are advanced to the full liquid diet next, adding bland and protein foods. A soft diet comes next, which omits foods that are hard to chew or digest. A regular or general diet has no limitations. A fluid restriction is ordered in addition to the diet order for clients in renal failure or congestive heart failure.

CN: Physiological integrity; CNS: Basic care and comfort; CL: Application

2. 3. The client's total intake is 1,330 ml. Use the following equation:

$$180 + 60 + 240 + 800 + 50 = 1,330.$$

CN: Physiological integrity; CNS: Basic care and comfort; CL: Analysis

3. 4. Each state has a Nurse Practice Act that dictates a nurse's scope of practice. Each nurse must practice competent standards based on her state's Nurse Practice Act. The ANA is an organization of nurses that offers credentialing and nursing education. It doesn't set standards of nursing practice. Physicians and pharmacists must practice competency based on the standards established by their professional organizations.

CN: Safe, effective care environment; CNS: Management of care; CL: Application

CN: Client needs category   CNS: Client needs subcategory   TL: Cognitive level

4. In checking a client's chart, the nurse notes that there's no record of an opioid being given to the client even though the previous nurse signed for one. The client denies receiving anything for pain since the previous night. Which action should be taken next?
    1. Notify the physician that an opioid is missing.
    2. Notify the supervisor that the client didn't receive the prescribed pain medication.
    3. Notify the pharmacist that the client didn't receive the prescribed pain medication.
    4. Approach the nurse who signed out the opioid to seek clarification about the missing drug.

5. A client is seen in the emergency department with bruises on her face and back. She has the signs of a domestic abuse victim. Which community resource could provide assistance to the client?
    1. Alcoholics Anonymous (AA)
    2. Crime Task Force
    3. Lifeline Emergency Aid
    4. Women's shelter

6. Multidisciplinary team meetings are used frequently as a method of communication among health care disciplines. Which unit uses this method of communication?
    1. Hemodialysis
    2. Home health care services
    3. Labor and delivery units
    4. Outpatient surgical units

7. A nurse finds a client crying after she was told hemodialysis is needed due to the development of acute renal failure. Which intervention is best?
    1. Sit quietly with the client.
    2. Refer the client to the hemodialysis team.
    3. Remind the client this is a temporary situation.
    4. Discuss with the client the other abilities she has.

4. 4. The nurse needs to seek clarification in a nonthreatening manner. If the nurse who signed out the opioid can't give a plausible explanation, the nurse who discovered the error must then notify the supervisor. The nurse who signed out the opioid may have a drug problem. The appropriate line of communication is to the hospital supervisor. The physician needs to be notified if the client didn't receive the prescribed medication. The pharmacist needs to be notified of discrepancies in the opioid count.
CN: Safe, effective care environment; CNS: Management of care; CL: Application

5. 4. A women's shelter can house women and children who need protection from an abusive partner or parent. AA is a support group for alcoholics and their families. The Crime Task Force and Lifeline Emergency Aid don't provide housing for women or children who want to leave an abusive relationship.
CN: Safe, effective care environment; CNS: Management of care; CL: Application

6. 2. Home health care services and restorative care services (such as rehabilitation units) that use different disciplines are required by The Joint Commission or Medicare to hold multidisciplinary team meetings. This serves as a means of communicating the client's diagnosis, plan of care, and discharge needs, using all disciplines for input. Hemodialysis units, outpatient surgical units, and labor and delivery units use between-shift reporting as a method of communicating and communicate among disciplines on an as needed basis.
CN: Safe, effective care environment; CNS: Management of care; CL: Application

7. 1. Sitting with the client shows compassion and concern, and may help the nurse establish therapeutic communication. Making a referral doesn't allow the client to explore feelings with the nurse. The nurse can't guarantee the acute renal failure is temporary. Discussing the client's other abilities is diverting the emphasis away from the primary issue for this client.
CN: Psychosocial integrity; CNS: None; CL: Analysis

8. A client was admitted to a mental health ward for hyperexcitability, increasing agitation, and distractibility. Which nursing intervention has priority?

 1. Involve the client in a group activity.
 2. Be direct, firm, and set rules for the client.
 3. Use a quiet room for the client away from others.
 4. Channel the client's energy toward a planned activity.

9. After maxillofacial surgery, a client, awake and alert, complains of pain, rating it as a 9 on a scale of 1 to 10. He receives meperidine (Demerol) 50 mg and hydroxyzine (Vistaril) 50 mg as ordered, every 4 hours as needed. Twenty minutes after the first dose, he reports his pain as a 6; 2 hours later, it's an 8. What might the nurse suspect is occurring?

 1. The hydroxyzine has interfered with the analgesic effect of the meperidine.
 2. The client has been moving too much.
 3. The client may need a higher dose.
 4. The prescription should be changed.

10. A public health nurse visiting a new postpartum client notices that the client has two children under age 4. The nurse notices one infant playing in the cabinet under the sink. Which instruction should the public health nurse give the client?

 1. Cover the infant's hands with gloves.
 2. Make sure all liquid cleaners are labeled.
 3. Tighten all cap tops on the bottles under the sink.
 4. Remove all cleaners that could be ingested orally.

11. A nurse arrives at a motor vehicle collision involving a school bus and a large truck. The school bus is lying on its side. Several people have been thrown from the windows of the school bus. Which victim needs priority care?

 1. A girl crying hysterically
 2. A boy who's unconscious
 3. A boy with a laceration of the scalp
 4. A girl with an obvious open fracture

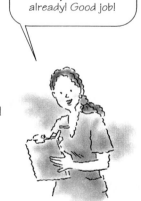

You've finished 10 questions already! Good job!

8. 3. Being in a quiet environment away from stimuli facilitates helping the client regain a sense of control. If the nurse attempts to be firm and set rules for this client, it will most likely heighten the agitation. The client is too excited to focus at this time; group activities or other activities may worsen the client's situation.
CN: Psychosocial integrity; CNS: None; CL: Application

9. 3. It's reasonable to assume that the dose is probably too low for the amount of pain, and it would be prudent to report the client's response to the physician and inquire if the physician feels it's appropriate to increase the dose. The hydroxyzine potentiates the effects of meperidine and doesn't interfere with its effectiveness. There's no evidence to suggest that the client has been moving around too much. It's beyond the nurse's scope of practice to determine that the current medication should be changed.
CN: Physiological integrity; CNS: Pharmacological and parenteral therapies; CL: Analysis

10. 4. All liquid cleaners must be removed to reduce the risk for poisoning. Safety locks should be placed on cabinets to prevent young children from opening the cabinets or the bottles. Infants can't read danger labels.
CN: Safe, effective care environment; CNS: Safety and infection control; CL: Application

11. 2. The unconscious child should be assessed for breathing and circulation status. An unconscious or unresponsive client always needs assistance first. Once help arrives, emotional support can be given to the girl crying hysterically, pressure can be applied to the laceration of the scalp to stop the bleeding, and the girl's fracture can be stabilized.
CN: Safe, effective care environment; CNS: Management of care; CL: Application

CN: Client needs category   CNS: Client needs subcategory   CL: Cognitive level

12. Which statement from a newly diagnosed client with diabetes indicates more instruction is needed?
   1. "I need to check my feet daily for sores."
   2. "I need to store my insulin in the refrigerator."
   3. "I can use my plastic insulin syringe more than once."
   4. "I need to see my physician for follow-up examinations."

13. A client with terminal cancer is receiving large doses of opioids for pain control. He becomes agitated and continues trying to get out of bed but can't stand without two-person assistance. To reduce the risk of falling, which type of restraint is the most beneficial?
   1. Leg restraints
   2. Chemical restraints
   3. Mechanical restraints
   4. Tying him in bed with a sheet

14. A client who had a stem cell transplant is in reverse isolation postoperatively. Which explanation for this precaution is correct?
   1. To protect the client from his own bacteria
   2. To protect the hospital staff from the client
   3. To protect the other clients on the nursing unit
   4. To protect the client from outside infections from others

15. A physician ordered a sterile dressing tray set up in a client's room to insert a subclavian central venous catheter. Which step is done first to set up the sterile field?
   1. Open the tray toward the nurse.
   2. Use correct handwashing technique.
   3. Put on sterile gloves before opening the tray.
   4. Place the sterile dressing tray on an overbed table.

12. 2. Insulin only needs to be stored in the refrigerator if it won't be used within 6 weeks after being opened; it should be at room temperature when given to decrease pain and prevent lipodystrophy. According to a poll by the Juvenile Diabetes Foundation, a very high percentage of diabetics reuse their insulin syringes. However, it's recommended they be carefully recapped and placed in the refrigerator to prevent bacterial growth. The remaining statements show that the client understands his condition and the importance of preventing complications.
CN: Safe, effective care environment; CNS: Safety and infection control; CL: Analysis

13. 2. Antianxiety medication can be used to calm the client. Chemical restraints are effective, especially with highly agitated clients receiving large doses of opioids. Other forms of restraint will only increase the client's agitation and hostility, thus increasing the safety risk.
CN: Safe, effective care environment; CNS: Safety and infection control; CL: Application

14. 4. Immunosuppressed clients need to be protected from infections from others following a stem cell transplant. Infections can occur if strict handwashing techniques aren't observed, especially with hospital staff going from one room to the next. Protective isolation is used to protect the hospital staff and other clients from an infected client.
CN: Safe, effective care environment; CNS: Safety and infection control; CL: Application

15. 2. Use appropriate handwashing technique before participating in a sterile procedure. Clean the area with an appropriate antiseptic, place the tray in the center of the clean area, and open it away from the nurse. After the dressing tray is opened, put on sterile gloves to assist the physician.
CN: Safe, effective care environment; CNS: Safety and infection control; CL: Application

16. Which action is included in the principles of asepsis?
1. Maintaining a sterile environment
2. Keeping the environment as clean as possible
3. Testing for microorganisms in the environment
4. Cleaning an environment until it's free from germs

17. A public health nurse is interviewing a young Pakistani client in her home. The nurse notices the client and the infant wear long skirts and coverings over their heads. The home isn't air-conditioned and the room is very warm. The dress code is recognized as part of which characteristic?
1. Culture
2. Economic status
3. Race
4. Socialization

18. A nurse is preparing a care plan for a client. Which action should be included in the assessment step of the nursing process?
1. Identify actual or potential health problems specific to the individual client.
2. Judge the effectiveness of nursing interventions that have been implemented.
3. Identify goals and interventions specific to the individualized needs of the client.
4. Systematically collect subjective and objective data with the goal of making a clinical nursing judgment.

19. During an interdepartmental team meeting at a hospice, a nurse who practices Catholicism verbalizes concern for the spiritual needs of a terminally ill infant and her non-Catholic family. She suggests the infant be baptized before death. Which recommendation of the multidisciplinary team is most likely?
1. Insist the infant obtain baptism before death occurs.
2. Bathe the infant with special oil to prepare for death.
3. Schedule an appointment with a Catholic priest to see the family.
4. Recognize that not all religions practice infant baptism.

16. 2. Asepsis is the process of avoiding contamination from outside sources by keeping the environment clean. A clean environment has a reduced number of microorganisms, but isn't necessarily sterile (the absence of all microorganisms). Testing for microorganisms or culturing isn't indicated in the promotion of asepsis.
CN; Safe, effective care environment; CNS: Safety and infection control; CL: Application

17. 1. Many cultures have specific dress codes. The client's dress, as described, doesn't indicate economic status. Race refers to a group of people with similar physical characteristics such as skin color. Socialization is the process by which individuals learn the ways of a given society to function within that group.
CN: Health promotion and maintenance; CNS: None; CL: Application

18. 4. Assessment involves data collection, organization, and validation. The diagnosis step of the nursing process involves the identification of actual or potential health problems. Evaluation involves judging the effectiveness of nursing interventions and whether the goals of the plan of care have been achieved. The nurse and client work together to identify goals, outcomes, and intervention strategies that will reduce identified client problems in the planning step.
CN: Safe, effective care environment; CNS: Management of care; CL: Application

19. 4. Many religious organizations (for example, Baptist, Adventist, Buddhist, Quaker) don't practice baptism or only baptize an individual when he or she is an adult. Hospice organizations use the family's religious leader as a choice for spiritual directions. Deciding whether to baptize the infant isn't the nurse's responsibility. Seventh Day Adventists believe in divine healing and anointing with oil. It's important to honor all customs and religious beliefs of families.
CN: Safe, effective care environment; CNS: Management of care; CL: Application

CN: Client needs category   CNS: Client needs subcategory   CL: Cognitive level

20. A home health client asks a nurse for information on sources of financial support. The client has an elderly parent who's blind living with her. Which program is the client referred to?
1. Medicare
2. Meals On Wheels
3. Supplemental Security Income
4. Aid to Families with Dependent Children

21. Giving hearing and vision screening to elementary school children is an example of which type of prevention strategy?
1. Primary
2. Secondary
3. Tertiary
4. None of the above

22. Which nursing action is most appropriate in relieving pain related to cancer?
1. Use heat or cold on painful areas.
2. Keep a hard bedroll behind the client's back.
3. Allow the client to stay in one position to prevent pain.
4. Keep bright lights on in the room so the nurse can assess the client more quickly.

23. A new graduate is assigned to a nursing unit. A nurse manager assesses that the graduate's skills are deficient. Which action is the most appropriate for the nurse manager to take?
1. Talk with the supervisor about terminating the new graduate.
2. Discuss with the graduate that a transfer to another unit is necessary.
3. Work with the graduate and develop a plan to improve the graduate's deficiencies.
4. Counsel the graduate that, if performance doesn't improve, the graduate will be terminated.

Stay focused, now. You're nearly one-third finished!

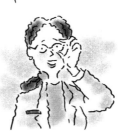

20. 3. Supplemental Security Income is a governmental subsidy assisting the poor and medically disabled. Medicare is available to elderly individuals age 65 years and older and individuals younger than 65 years with long-term disabilities or end-stage renal disease. Meals On Wheels is a nonprofit organization that delivers food to the poor. Aid to Families with Dependent Children is a state subsidy given to poor families with dependent children.
CN: Safe, effective care environment; CNS: Management of care; CL: Application

21. 2. Screening is a major secondary prevention strategy. Secondary prevention is aimed at early detection and treatment of illness. Primary prevention strategies are aimed at preventing the disease from the beginning by avoiding or modifying risk factors. Tertiary prevention strategies focus on rehabilitation and prevention of complications arising from advanced disease.
CN: Health promotion and maintenance; CNS: None; CL: Application

22. 1. Using either heat or cold can reduce inflammatory responses, which will reduce pain. Avoid pressure (such as bedrolls) on painful areas. Change the client's position frequently. Coordinate activity with pain medication. Reduce bright lights and noise to prevent anxiety, which can increase pain.
CN: Physiological integrity; CNS: Physiological adaptation; CL: Application

23. 3. The leader needs to work with the new graduate and provide opportunities for the graduate to grow and develop. The other responses wouldn't give the new graduate the opportunity and support needed for improvement.
CN: Safe, effective care environment; CNS: Management of care; CL: Application

24. A local community health nurse is asked to speak to a group of adolescent girls on the topic of preventing pregnancy. Which statement indicates the adolescents need more information on this topic?
1. "I can get pregnant even on the first time we have sex."
2. "I can get pregnant even though I don't have sex regularly."
3. "I can't get pregnant because my menstrual cycle isn't regular yet."
4. "I can get pregnant even if my boyfriend withdraws before he comes."

24. 3. Many adolescents have misunderstandings related to risk periods and timing, including periods of susceptibility during the menstrual cycle, age-related susceptibility, and timing of male ejaculation.
CN: Health promotion and maintenance; CNS: None; CL: Analysis

25. Which nursing action is most appropriate in stimulating the appetite of a child with cancer?
1. Use food as a reward system.
2. Serve large meals frequently.
3. Prepare foods appropriate to the age of the child.
4. Place the child on a rigid time schedule for eating.

25. 3. It's important to prepare foods appropriate to children in certain age groups. Involve the child in food preparation and selection. Assess the family's beliefs about food habits. Let the child eat all food that can be tolerated. Take advantage of a hungry period and serve small snacks. Encourage parents to relax pressures placed on eating by stressing the legitimate nature of loss of appetite.
CN: Physiological integrity; CNS: Physiological adaptation; CL: Application

26. A nurse working in a public health clinic is planning tuberculosis (TB) screening. Screening is indicated for which group?
1. All clients coming into the clinic
2. People living in a homeless shelter
3. Clients who haven't received the TB vaccine
4. Clients suspected of having human immunodeficiency virus (HIV)

26. 4. Clients with HIV infection or suspected of having HIV are at greater risk for developing TB. A screening test should be done and, if positive, treatment with isoniazid (Nydrazid) given. Clients coming to the clinic don't need to be tested unless they're at high risk — for example, living with someone infected with TB, abusing I.V. drugs, or suffering from chronic health conditions, such as diabetes mellitus and end-stage renal disease. Clients living in a homeless shelter aren't necessarily at greater risk unless other residents in the shelter have TB. The TB vaccine isn't widely used in the United States.
CN: Health promotion and maintenance; CNS: None; CL: Application

27. A professional nurse should report positive tuberculosis (TB) smears or cultures to the health department within which time period?
1. 12 hours
2. 48 hours
3. 1 week
4. 10 to 14 days

27. 2. A client is considered contagious if he has a positive TB smear or culture, so the results must be reported within 24 to 48 hours. The smear or culture may not have grown an organism in 12 hours. One week or 10 to 14 days is too long to wait.
CN: Safe, effective care environment; CNS: Safety and infection control; CL: Application

CN: Client needs category   CNS: Client needs subcategory   CL: Cognitive level

28. A 62-year-old female client has been taking vitamin C 500 mg by mouth (P.O.) daily, multivitamins 1 tablet P.O. every day, and aspirin 325 mg every 6 hours as needed for arthritic pain for 4 days. The nurse notices that the client's stool is becoming darker and that a test for occult blood is positive. What would the nurse most likely conclude?

  1. The combination of vitamin C and multivitamins are irritating the lining of the intestine.
  2. The aspirin should be withheld because it may be causing gastric bleeding.
  3. Vitamin C is acidic in nature and may be irritating the GI tissues.
  4. From the appearance of the stool, the nurse suspects the client has hemorrhoids.

29. In which nurse-client interaction is a home health nurse demonstrating a secondary intervention as an advocate?

  1. Contacting the local church to borrow a walker for the client to use
  2. Listening to a client express feelings of frustration over the limitations imposed by his condition
  3. Giving I.V. antibiotic therapy every 12 hours with attention to sterile technique and prevention of complications
  4. Teaching a client with chronic obstructive pulmonary disease the effect of abdominal distention on breathing and ways to help bowel function

30. Which action is an example of indirect care function of a home health nurse?

  1. Supervising a home health aide
  2. Participating in a team conference about a client
  3. Showing the home health aide body positioning for the client
  4. Teaching the care provider how to read a food label for sodium content

31. A young pregnant client attending prenatal classes is concerned about her alcohol intake. Which statement indicates the client's child is at high risk of fetal alcohol syndrome (FAS)?

  1. "I just snort once or twice a day."
  2. "I had one glass of wine with dinner last week."
  3. "I drink a six pack of beer daily to settle my nerves."
  4. "I smoke marijuana with my boyfriend and his friends."

28. 2. Aspirin is widely known for causing gastric irritation and bleeding. Vitamin C and multivitamins generally don't have an adverse effect in the GI tract. There may be hemorrhoids present, but bleeding from this source would generally be bright red.

CN: Physiological integrity; CNS: Pharmacological and parenteral therapies; CL: Analysis

29. 1. Referral to community agencies is an advocacy role for home health nurses. The role of the advocate implies the home care nurse is able to advise clients how to find alternative sources of care. Giving emotional support, giving therapies to clients, and instructing clients about disease processes are direct care activities.

CN: Safe, effective care environment; CNS: Management of care; CL: Application

30. 2. Participating in a team conference is an example of indirect care. Direct care is defined as the actual nursing care given to clients in their homes. Direct care may involve assessment of physical or psychosocial status, performance of skilled interventions, supervision of other disciplines, and teaching.

CN: Safe, effective care environment; CNS: Management of care; CL: Application

31. 3. Ingestion of alcohol on a daily basis increases the risk of FAS. Other forms of addictive behavior, such as the ingestion of cocaine and smoking marijuana, increase the risk of fetal abuse—not fetal alcohol syndrome.

CN: Health promotion and maintenance; CNS: None; CL: Analysis

32. According to the Centers for Disease Control and Prevention, which group most likely would need preventive therapy for tuberculosis (TB)?
1. Clients with human immunodeficiency virus (HIV) infection
2. Clients with recent tuberculin skin tests and low risk
3. Persons with no contact with infectious TB clients
4. Clients with abnormal chest X-rays

33. Which psychosocial approach should an emergency department nurse use when dealing with suspected family violence?
1. Punitive
2. Supportive treatment
3. Disgust and avoidance
4. Get the facts at all costs

34. A concerned client called the school asking that the nurse assess her 13-year-old son for signs of depression. Which symptom should the nurse expect to see?
1. Becomes angry at peers easily
2. Seeks out support from peers
3. Eats several small meals daily
4. Feels he can control everything in his life

35. A 56-year-old client recently lost his 82-year-old father to lung cancer. In counseling the client, the bereavement nurse expects which sign of grief?
1. Decreased libido
2. Absence of anger and hostility
3. Difficulty crying or controlling crying
4. Clear dreams and imagery of the deceased

36. A 72-year-old client experienced the death of his wife 1 year ago. He now needs home health services due to severe osteoarthritis. Which statement indicates the client will need further bereavement counseling?
1. "I'm lucky my children live so close."
2. "I really don't have anything to live for."
3. "My health isn't very good, but I can live with it."
4. "I've always had trouble remembering where I placed things."

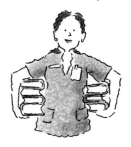

Didn't I tell you all your hard work would pay off?

32. 1. Preventive therapy should be initiated for clients infected with HIV because latent TB can become active if the immune system is weakened. Clients with low risk and negative skin tests are unlikely to be infected with TB or to progress if infected. Clients with no contact with infectious TB cases aren't at high risk for developing TB. Although clients with active TB may have abnormal chest X-rays, many other conditions can cause abnormalities.
CN: Health promotion and maintenance; CNS: None; CL: Application

33. 2. Emotional support is a nonthreatening approach when dealing with suspected family violence. Aggressive, punitive, and disdainful approaches can increase the anxiety of the perpetrator, increasing the risk of more violence.
CN: Psychosocial integrity; CNS: None; CL: Application

34. 1. Adolescents experiencing depression may experience and express anger at peers. Adolescents feel a lack of control over their current situation, so they isolate themselves from their peers. The adolescent often has an intake of nutrients insufficient to meet metabolic needs.
CN: Psychosocial integrity; CNS: None; CL: Analysis

35. 4. A grieving client usually has vivid, clear dreams and fantasies. He also has a good capacity for imagery, particularly involving the loss. Difficulty crying or controlling crying, absence of anger and hostility, and decreased libido are signs of depression.
CN: Psychosocial integrity; CNS: None; CL: Analysis

36. 2. Wishing for death is a sign of depression. Usually after a year, most individuals accept the death of their loved ones and begin restoring their lives. Being grateful for good health and close family ties is a sign of acceptance of a new life that one experiences after the loss of a loved one. Memory loss can be a sign of dementia or depression.
CN: Psychosocial integrity; CNS: None; CL: Analysis

CN: Client needs category   CNS: Client needs subcategory   CL: Cognitive level

37. A client in the second stage of labor reports strong urges to bear down. The nurse interprets this reflex as:
1. Babinski's reflex
2. Ferguson's reflex
3. Moro's reflex
4. Myerson's reflex

38. Which nursing action is most appropriate for handling chemotherapeutic agents?
1. Wear disposable gloves and protective clothing.
2. Break needles after the infusion is discontinued.
3. Disconnect I.V. tubing with gloved hands.
4. Throw I.V. tubing in the trash after the infusion is discontinued.

39. A client developed oral ulcerations secondary to chemotherapy agents. Which nursing action is most appropriate for reducing pain and irritation in the mouth?
1. Serve a high-fiber diet.
2. Use a toothbrush to clean teeth.
3. Avoid taking oral temperatures.
4. Rinse the mouth with hydrogen peroxide and water.

40. A client is admitted to the emergency department after being sexually assaulted. Which nursing intervention receives priority?
1. Assisting with medical treatment
2. Collecting and preparing evidence for the police
3. Attempting to reduce the client's anxiety from a panic to a moderate level
4. Providing anticipatory guidance to the client about normal responses to sexual assault

37. 2. Ferguson's reflex is characterized by the strong urge to bear down during the second stage of labor. Babinski's reflex results in dorsiflexion of the big toe and fanning of the other toes when the sole of a client's foot is scraped. Moro's reflex is a normal generalized reflex in an infant when he reacts to a sudden noise, such as when a table next to him is struck. Myerson's reflex results in blinking when the client's forehead, bridge of the nose, or maxilla is tapped.
CN: Physiological integrity; CNS: Physiological adaptation; CL: Analysis

38. 1. A nurse must wear disposable gloves and protective clothing to protect skin contact with the chemotherapeutic agent. Don't recap or break needles. Use a sterile gauze pad when priming I.V. tubing, connecting and disconnecting tubing, inserting syringes into vials, breaking glass ampules, or other procedures in which chemotherapeutic agents are being handled. Contaminated needles, syringes, I.V. tubes, and other contaminated equipment must be disposed of in a leak-proof, puncture-resistant container.
CN: Physiological integrity; CNS: Pharmacological and parenteral therapies; CL: Application

39. 3. If oral ulcers are present, taking oral temperatures will be painful. Use the axillary region, rectum, or ear as sites for temperature readings. Serving a high-fiber diet won't reduce mouth pain and irritation. Use a soft-sponge toothbrush, cotton-tipped applicator, or gauze-wrapped finger to clean teeth. Give normal saline solution mouthwashes and rinses to reduce pain and inflammation. Hydrogen peroxide mixed with water is too irritating if oral ulcers are present.
CN: Physiological integrity; CNS: Basic care and comfort; CL: Application

40. 3. Reducing anxiety will help the client participate in medical, forensic, and legal follow-up activities. Medical treatment should begin as soon as the client's anxiety decreases below the panic level. Collecting and preparing evidence and providing anticipatory guidance aren't high-priority interventions.
CN: Psychosocial integrity; CNS: None; CL: Analysis

41. The nurse is caring for an 8-year-old boy diagnosed with attention deficit hyperactivity disorder (ADHD). Which behavior is the nurse most likely to observe in this client?
   1. Lethargy
   2. Long attention span
   3. Short attention span
   4. Preoccupation with body parts

42. A client with burns on 50% of his body is receiving total parenteral nutrition (TPN). Which symptom indicates the client is having a complication of TPN?
   1. Pain
   2. Absent bowel sounds
   3. Abdominal cramping
   4. Increased urine glucose

43. A 35-year-old client is admitted to an inpatient substance abuse unit with a diagnosis of alcohol dependence. Which comment by the client supports this diagnosis?
   1. "I don't drink more than two beers when I'm out."
   2. "I always remember what happens the next day."
   3. "I always ask a friend to drive me home when I'm drinking."
   4. "I've had four tickets for driving while intoxicated last month."

44. A nurse is working with a client with alcoholism in an acute care mental health unit. The client has been referred to Alcoholics Anonymous (AA). Which statement best indicates that the client is ready to begin the AA program?
   1. "I know I'm powerless over alcohol and need help."
   2. "I think it will be interesting and helpful to join AA."
   3. "I'd like to sponsor another alcoholic with this same problem."
   4. "My family is very supportive and will attend meetings with me."

41. 3. Short attention span is a common characteristic of ADHD due to difficulty concentrating. These children show hyperexcitability, not lethargy. Children with this disorder are distracted by environmental stimuli, so they won't be concentrating on their body parts.
CN: Psychosocial integrity; CNS: None; CL: Application

42. 4. Glycosuria, increased urine glucose, is associated with high blood glucose levels, a complication of TPN. Pain from major burns is expected. Absent bowel sounds are an indication to begin TPN. Abdominal cramping is associated with diarrhea or constipation.
CN: Physiological integrity; CNS: Basic care and comfort; CL: Application

43. 4. Driving while intoxicated can be seen as a symptom of alcohol dependence. Designating drivers and limiting alcohol consumption are self-responsible actions, but don't address the underlying problem. The amount one drinks doesn't matter. An alcoholic experiences blackouts, which are periods of amnesia about experiences while intoxicated. By asking someone to drive them home, clients with alcohol dependence rationalize that it's okay to drink if they're responsible.
CN: Psychosocial integrity; CNS: None; CL: Analysis

44. 1. In step 1 of AA, a person admits his powerlessness over alcohol and is ready to accept help. This should occur before he begins AA. A supportive family and a desire to help others with the same problem are good for the client, but they don't necessarily indicate readiness to participate in the program.
CN: Psychosocial integrity; CNS: None; CL: Application

CN: Client needs category   CNS: Client needs subcategory   CL: Cognitive level

45. In planning care for a client diagnosed with paranoid schizophrenia, which action is correct for the psychiatric home health nurse?
 1. Confront the client about her hallucinations.
 2. Ask the minister to provide spiritual direction.
 3. Instruct family members to discourage delusions.
 4. Affirm when the client's perceptions and thinking are in touch with reality.

45. 4. The nursing plan of care focuses on reinforcing perceptions and thinking that are in touch with reality. Confronting a client about her hallucinations and delusions isn't effective or therapeutic. Spiritual direction is important, but a client with paranoid schizophrenia may have issues surrounding her religious or spiritual orientation. Therefore, asking a minister to provide spiritual direction may not be effective or therapeutic. Using family members could create distrust between the client and the family.
CN: Psychosocial integrity; CNS: None; CL: Application

46. A psychiatric home health nurse finds a client with bipolar disorder sitting on the porch. The client is wearing a red polka dot dress, large yellow hat, and heavy makeup with large gold jewelry. Which phase of the illness is the client most likely in?
 1. Delusional
 2. Depressive
 3. Manic
 4. Suspicious

46. 3. Extreme labile moods are characteristic of clients in the manic phase of bipolar disorder. Hyperactivity, verbosity, and drawing attention to oneself through dress are typical of the manic phase. Delusions and suspiciousness may be seen in bipolar disorder, but are more commonly seen in schizophrenia. In the depressive phase, clients are withdrawn, cry, and may not eat. Visual or auditory hallucinations, delusional thoughts, and extreme suspiciousness are behaviors seen in clients diagnosed with paranoid schizophrenia.
CN: Psychosocial integrity; CNS: None; CL: Analysis

47. A nurse is assessing a 4-week-old neonate for signs of acute pain. Which symptom is expected?
 1. Whimpering
 2. Eyes opened wide
 3. Limp body posture
 4. Wanting to breast-feed frequently

47. 1. Crying, whimpering, and groaning are vocal expressions of acute pain in the neonate. Eyes tightly closed, changes in feeding behavior, and fist clenching with rigidity also are signs of acute pain in the neonate.
CN: Health promotion and maintenance; CNS: None; CL: Application

48. A home health nurse is instructing a client about positioning her child, who's diagnosed with juvenile rheumatoid arthritis (JRA). Which position or equipment is needed to maintain posture for a child with JRA?
 1. Soft mattress
 2. Prone position
 3. Large fluffy pillows
 4. Semi-Fowler's position

48. 2. Lying in the prone position is encouraged to straighten hips and knees. A firm mattress is needed to maintain good alignment of spine, hips, and knees, and no pillow or a very thin pillow should be used. Semi-Fowler's position increases pressure on the hip joints and should be avoided.
CN: Physiological integrity; CNS: Basic care and comfort; CL: Application

49. Which comfort measure is best to reduce pain and stiffness for a child with juvenile rheumatoid arthritis (JRA)?
1. Hot packs
2. Cool baths
3. Cold compresses
4. Immersion in lukewarm water for 10 minutes

50. While putting an elderly client with an indwelling urinary catheter in bed, the nurse places the tubing in a loop on the bed with the client and makes sure the client won't lie on the tubing. Which rationale explains the nurse's action?
1. To inhibit drainage
2. To allow drainage to occur
3. To allow the urine to collect in the tubing
4. To have the client check the tubing for urine

51. A client complains of severe burning on urination. Which instruction is best to give the client?
1. Wear only nylon underwear.
2. Drink coffee to increase urination.
3. Soak in warm water with bubble bath.
4. Drink 2,500 to 3,000 ml of water per day.

52. Which instruction is given to a client with a hearing aid?
1. Clean the hearing aid with baby oil.
2. Wear the hearing aid while sleeping.
3. Keep the hearing aid out of direct sunlight.
4. Leave the hearing aid in place while showering.

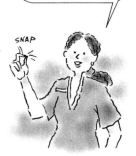

You've finished 50 questions! The remaining 25 should be a snap!

SNAP

49. 1. Heat is beneficial to children with arthritis. Moist heat is best for relieving pain and stiffness. The most efficient and practical method is in the bathtub. Cold, cool, or luke-warm treatment isn't beneficial in relieving pain or stiffness in children with JRA.
CN: Physiological integrity; CNS: Basic care and comfort; CL: Application

50. 2. Catheter tubing shouldn't be allowed to develop dependent loops or kinks because this inhibits proper drainage by requiring the urine to travel against gravity to empty into the bag. Permitting the urine to collect in the tubing increases the risk of infection. Observing the catheter and tubing is the responsibility of the nurse.
CN: Physiological integrity; CNS: Reduction of risk potential; CL: Application

51. 4. Drinking large amounts of water will help flush bacteria from the urinary tract. Avoid nylon underwear; wear only cotton undergarments to decrease the warm, moist environment. Avoid tea, coffee, carbonated drinks, and alcoholic beverages because of bladder irritation. Avoid using bubble baths, perfumed soaps, or bath powders in the perineal area. The scent in toiletries can be irritating to the urinary meatus.
CN: Physiological integrity; CNS: Basic care and comfort; CL: Application

52. 3. The hearing aid should be kept out of direct sunlight and away from high temperatures. Solvents or lubricants shouldn't be used on the aid. If there is a detachable ear mold, it can be washed in warm, soapy water and dried with a soft cloth. The hearing aid should be left in place while the client is awake, except when showering.
CN: Physiological integrity; CNS: Basic care and comfort; CL: Application

CN: Client needs category   CNS: Client needs subcategory   CL: Cognitive level

53. A 72-year-old client is being discharged from same-day surgery after having a cataract removed from his right eye. Which discharge instruction does a nurse give the client?

1. Sleep on the operative side.
2. Resume all activities as before.
3. Don't rub or place pressure on the eyes.
4. Wear an eye shield all day and remove it at night.

54. To ensure the safe administration of medications, which action should be performed first?

1. Make sure the client is in the correct room.
2. Check for client allergies.
3. Have the client repeat his name.
4. Open the medications at the client's bedside.

55. Which instruction is correct for a client taking nortriptyline (Pamelor) for depression?

1. Be aware that this drug can cause hypotension.
2. This drug will work immediately to treat depression.
3. Take this drug in the morning because it causes drowsiness.
4. Wear protective clothing and sunscreen when out in the sun.

56. Which instruction is correct for a client receiving lithium (Eskalith) for bipolar disorder?

1. Avoid drugs containing ibuprofen.
2. Drink at least two cups of coffee daily.
3. Be aware that you may experience increased alertness.
4. It isn't necessary to monitor the blood level of this drug.

53. 3. Rubbing or placing pressure on the eyes increases the risk of accidental injury to ocular structures. The nurse should also caution against lifting objects, straining, strenuous exercise, and sexual activity because such activities can increase intraocular pressure. Caution against sleeping on the operative side to reduce the risk of accidental injury to ocular structures. Glasses or shaded lenses should be worn to protect the eye during waking hours after the eye dressing is removed. An eye shield should be worn at night.

CN: Physiological integrity; CNS: Reduction of risk potential; CL: Application

54. 2. Checking for client allergies is the first step in ensuring safe administration of medications. The other actions are important, but not the priority.

CN: Physiological integrity; CNS: Pharmacological and parenteral therapies; CL: Analysis

55. 4. A common adverse effect of this drug is sensitivity to the sun. Protective clothing and sunscreen are worn in the sun. This drug can cause hypertension. It doesn't work immediately, but takes 2 to 3 weeks to achieve the desired effect. This drug should be taken at bedtime if it causes drowsiness.

CN: Physiological integrity; CNS: Pharmacological and parenteral therapies; CL: Application

56. 1. Avoid drugs that alter the effect of lithium, such as ibuprofen and sodium bicarbonate or other antacids containing sodium. Avoid beverages with caffeine because they increase urination, which may alter the effect of lithium. Lithium can decrease alertness and coordination. Lithium levels may need to be monitored every 2 weeks, especially if adverse effects occur. The dose may need to be regulated.

CN: Physiological integrity; CNS: Pharmacological and parenteral therapies; CL: Application

57. A physician ordered nitroprusside I.V. for a client in cardiogenic shock. Which nursing intervention is needed to give this drug safely?
  1. Give only with other drugs.
  2. Mix the drug in an alkaline solution.
  3. Mix the drug only in normal saline solution.
  4. Cover the drug-containing I.V. solution with an opaque wrapper.

58. Which nursing intervention is correct for a client receiving total parenteral nutrition (TPN)?
  1. Discard TPN solutions after 24 hours.
  2. Discard lipid emulsions after 20 hours.
  3. Inspect the TPN solution for clearness and visibility.
  4. Teach the client to blow out during expiration when the tubing is disconnected.

59. Which opioid analgesic may be given parenterally to an older client to be more useful?
  1. Hydromorphone (Dilaudid)
  2. Meperidine (Demerol)
  3. Morphine
  4. Oxycodone (Percocet)

60. Which diagnostic test is used to diagnose bacterial endocarditis?
  1. Electrolytes
  2. Blood cultures
  3. Prothrombin time (PT)
  4. Venereal Disease Research Laboratory (VDRL)

57. 4. The nurse should cover the drug-containing I.V. solution with an opaque wrapper because the drug is light-sensitive. Nitroprusside can't be mixed in alkaline solutions, and shouldn't be given with other drugs. Only dilute the drug in dextrose 5% in water; no other fluid should be used.
CN: Physiological integrity; CNS: Pharmacological and parenteral therapies; CL: Application

58. 1. TPN solutions are good media for fungi, so they should be discarded after 24 hours. Lipid emulsions are also good media for fungi and should be discarded after 12 hours. Inspect TPN solutions for cloudiness, cracks, or leaks before hanging. The nurse should teach the client to perform Valsalva's maneuver, taking a deep breath and holding it, when the tubing is disconnected. Valsalva's maneuver increases intrathoracic pressure, which prevents air entry.
CN: Physiological integrity; CNS: Pharmacological and parenteral therapies; CL: Application

59. 1. Hydromorphone is a fast-acting drug and is a useful alternative to morphine or meperidine due to its short half-life. Morphine and meperidine can increase the risk of confusion in the elderly. Oxycodone is given only orally or rectally.
CN: Physiological integrity; CNS: Pharmacological and parenteral therapies; CL: Application

60. 2. Blood cultures are crucial in diagnosing bacterial endocarditis. Electrolyte levels indicate abnormalities that occur with drug therapy as well as with complications associated with heart failure. PT values are useful in monitoring anticoagulant therapy. A positive VDRL may be evidence of syphilitic heart disease.
CN: Physiological integrity; CNS: Reduction of risk potential; CL: Application

CN: Client needs category   CNS: Client needs subcategory   CL: Cognitive level

61. In preparing a client for cardiac catheterization, which statement or question is most appropriate?
1. "Are you allergic to contrast dyes or shellfish?"
2. "Have you ever had this kind of procedure before?"
3. "You'll need to fast 24 hours before the procedure."
4. "You'll be given medication to help you sleep during the procedure."

61. 1. The nurse must assess the client for allergies to iodine before the procedure because the dye used during catheterization contains iodine. Knowing the client's history and prior experience with this procedure would be helpful, but knowing the client's allergies is more important. The client is instructed to fast for 6 hours before the procedure. The client will be asked to empty his bladder before the procedure. The client needs to stay awake during the procedure to follow directions, such as taking a deep breath and holding it during injection of the dye, and to report chest, neck, or jaw discomfort.
CN: Physiological integrity; CNS: Reduction of risk potential; CL: Application

62. A 60-year-old male client is suspected of having coronary artery disease. Which noninvasive diagnostic method would the nurse expect to be ordered to evaluate cardiac changes?
1. Cardiac biopsy
2. Cardiac catheterization
3. Magnetic resonance imaging (MRI)
4. Pericardiocentesis

62. 3. MRI is a noninvasive procedure that aids in the diagnosis and detection of thoracic aortic aneurysm and evaluation of coronary artery disease, pericardial disease, and cardiac masses. Cardiac biopsy, cardiac catheterization, and pericardiocentesis are invasive techniques used to evaluate cardiac changes.
CN: Health promotion and maintenance; CNS: None; CL: Application

63. In evaluating an electrocardiogram (ECG) strip in a telemetry unit, a nurse notices a client is having premature ventricular contractions (PVCs). Which criteria is used to evaluate the presence of PVCs on the ECG strip?
1. There's no PR interval.
2. The R-R interval is irregular.
3. Ventricular rate is slower than atrial rate.
4. The QRS complex is followed by a compensatory pause.

63. 4. The QRS complex is followed by a compensatory pause that ends when the underlying rhythm resumes. This is one of the ECG criteria used to evaluate PVCs. The remaining responses are ECG criteria used to evaluate atrial flutter.
CN: Physiological integrity; CNS: Reduction of risk potential; CL: Analysis

64. In evaluating an electrocardiogram (ECG) strip for the presence of a pacemaker, which criteria indicates a malfunction?
1. Short T waves
2. Normal sinus rhythm
3. Pacing spikes appearing at different times during a cardiac cycle
4. Pacing spike followed by a wide QRS complex

64. 3. When pacing spikes appear at different times during a cardiac cycle, it indicates a failure to capture. Failure to capture may result in inappropriate pacing; the ECG would show a pacing spike delivered on time but not followed by a wide QRS complex. Tall T waves or an irregular heart rate indicate a failure-to-sense malfunction.
CN: Physiological integrity; CNS: Reduction of risk potential; CL: Analysis

65. In caring for a client with arterial insufficiency, which instruction is most appropriate for home health teaching?
1. "You may leave your feet open to the air."
2. "It's best to sit and rest for several hours a day."
3. "Avoid crossing your legs at the knees or ankles."
4. "It's best to wear tight socks instead of no socks."

66. Which instruction is correct for home health teaching for a client taking oral anticoagulants?
1. "You may shave with a standard razor."
2. "You may take ibuprofen or aspirin for pain."
3. "Take the anticoagulant at the same time each day."
4. "It's important to eat a large quantity of green, leafy vegetables."

67. Which action is most appropriate to reduce sensory deprivation for a visually impaired elderly client in the hospital?
1. Keep the lights dimmed.
2. Close the curtains or blinds on windows to reduce glare.
3. Open the hospital door so bright light can shine in the room.
4. Open the curtains during the day so the sun can shine brightly.

68. Which action is most appropriate to reduce sensory overload for a hearing-impaired elderly client in the coronary care unit?
1. Keep the overhead light on continuously.
2. Discuss the client's condition at the bedside.
3. Allow all family members to stay with the client.
4. Limit bedside conversation to that directed to the client.

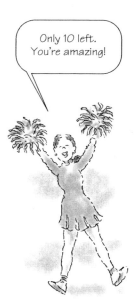

Only 10 left. You're amazing!

65. 3. Leg crossing should be avoided because it compresses the vessels in the legs. Feet and extremities must be protected to reduce the risk of trauma. Sitting for several hours isn't recommended. Avoid constrictive clothing, such as tight elastic on socks, to prevent compression of vessels in the legs.
CN: Physiological integrity; CNS: Reduction of risk potential; CL: Application

66. 3. It's important to take the anticoagulant at the same time each day to maintain an adequate blood level. An electric razor reduces the risk of cutting the skin. Avoid the use of standard razors. Avoid taking aspirin or ibuprofen because these drugs decrease clotting time. Eating a large amount of green, leafy vegetables, which contain vitamin K, increases the clotting time, thus requiring more anticoagulants.
CN: Physiological integrity; CNS: Pharmacological and parenteral therapies; CL: Application

67. 2. Closing curtains or blinds on windows can reduce glare and improve vision for the older client. Controlled lighting can help the older client see better in the hospital. Adequate background lighting helps the older client decrease visual accommodation when moving from brightly lit to dimly lit rooms and hallways.
CN: Physiological integrity; CNS: Reduction of risk potential; CL: Application

68. 4. Limiting bedside conversation to that directed to the client creates fewer disturbances, thus reducing sensory overload. Turning off or dimming the overhead lights further reduces visual stimulation and facilitates day and night light fluctuations. Although fostering family interaction with the client is necessary, only one or two family members should be allowed to visit with the client at one time. Crowding of people in the client's room may precipitate a loss of privacy and control for the client.
CN: Physiological integrity; CNS: Reduction of risk potential; CL: Application

CN: Client needs category CNS: Client needs subcategory CL: Cognitive level

69. Which instruction is most appropriate in home health teaching for a client with osteoarthritis of the left knee?
1. Use cold on joints.
2. Keep the knee extended.
3. Maintain a healthy weight.
4. Have someone help the client in activities of daily living (ADL).

70. A home care aide notified the agency that she found a client lying on the floor. When the home health nurse arrives, the newly diagnosed diabetic client is semicomatose, with a fast heart rate and low blood pressure. The client's skin is warm and dry. Which condition is indicated?
1. Hypoglycemia
2. Cardiogenic shock
3. Diabetic ketoacidosis (DKA)
4. Hyperosmolar hypoglycemic nonketotic syndrome (HHNS)

71. A nurse is standing next to a person eating fried shrimp at a parade. Suddenly, the man clutches at his throat and is unable to speak, cough, or breathe. The nurse asks the man if he's choking and he nods yes. Which response is most appropriate?
1. Attempt rescue breathing.
2. Perform the Heimlich maneuver.
3. Deliver external chest compressions.
4. Use the head tilt-chin lift maneuver to establish the airway.

72. Which response is most appropriate to prepare for a cardiopulmonary emergency?
1. Have nasal oxygen ready when needed.
2. Place an oropharyngeal airway at the bedside.
3. Keep the medication cart locked up for safety.
4. Don't start an I.V. line unless necessary.

69. 3. Maintaining a healthy weight decreases joint stress. Local moist heat provides pain relief and will decrease stiffness. The client should perform muscle-strengthening exercises, which help prevent joint stiffness. The nurse should allow the client to perform ADL with less assistance.
CN: Physiological integrity; CNS: Reduction of risk potential; CL: Application

70. 3. DKA develops as a result of severe insulin deficiency. The incidence of DKA generally results from undiagnosed diabetes and inadequacy of prescribed medication and dietary therapies. Hypoglycemia involves episodes of low blood glucose levels caused by erratic or altered absorption of insulin. In cardiogenic shock, the client has pale, cool, and moist skin. HHNS is a deadly complication of diabetes distinguished by severe hyperglycemia, dehydration, and changed mental status.
CN: Physiological integrity; CNS: Physiological adaptation; CL: Application

71. 2. If a conscious victim acknowledges that he's choking, the best response is to perform the Heimlich maneuver to relieve the airway obstruction. The other options are used for an unresponsive victim with absent heart rate and breathing.
CN: Physiological integrity; CNS: Physiological adaptation; CL: Application

72. 2. A nurse should learn to anticipate clinical deterioration before overt signs and symptoms are apparent. If a client is having breathing difficulties, the nurse should place an oropharyngeal airway at the bedside while the client is monitored for deterioration. The emergency cart should be placed outside the client's room for easy access. If breathing stops, the client will need to be intubated and placed on a respirator, if necessary. The client should have a stable I.V. line for administration of emergency drugs.
CN: Physiological integrity; CNS: Physiological adaptation; CL: Analysis

73. In preparing for cardioversion, which action is most appropriate?
1. Keep the client awake and alert.
2. Keep the side rails up for client safety.
3. Set the machine on SYNC and charge at 200 watts.
4. Set the machine on DEFIB and charge at 400 watts.

74. A client who is at 37 weeks' gestation comes to the office for a prenatal visit. The nurse performs Leopold's maneuvers to assess the position of the fetus. After performing the maneuvers, the nurse suspects that the physician will attempt external version. Where did the nurse palpate the head of the fetus?

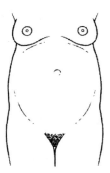

75. A physician orders an I.V. infusion of dextrose 5% in quarter-normal saline solution to be infused at 7 ml/kg/hour for a 10-month-old infant. The infant weighs 22 lb. How many ml/hour of the ordered solution should the nurse infuse? Record your answer using a whole number.

_____ milliliters/hour

73. 3. If cardioversion is needed, the nurse should set the machine on SYNC and look for a marker on each QRS complex. The nurse should start at a low energy level and increase as needed. The nurse should sedate the client and lower the side rails for easier placement of paddle electrodes.

CN: Physiological integrity; CNS: Physiological adaptation; CL: Application

74. If the fetal head is palpated at the top of the uterus, the fetus is in the breech position. The physician may consider external version to convert the fetus to a vertex lie, or head-down position. This is accomplished by applying pressure on the maternal abdomen to turn the infant over, as in a somersault.

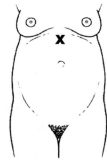

CN: Physiological integrity; CNS: Reduction of risk potential; CL: Analysis

75. 70. To perform this dosage calculation, the nurse should first convert the infant's weight to kilograms: 2.2 lb/kg = 22 lb/X kg; X = 22 ÷ 2.2; X = 10 kg. Next, she should multiply the infant's weight by the ordered rate: 10 kg × 7 ml/kg/hour = 70 ml/hour.

CN: Physiological integrity; CNS: Pharmacological and parenteral therapies; CL: Application

CN: Client needs category   CNS: Client needs subcategory   CL: Cognitive level

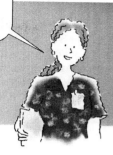

Here's another comprehensive test to help you get ready to take the NCLEX test. Good luck!

COMPREHENSIVE
Test 4

1. A nurse-manager has identified several personal problems with a staff member. Which approach is best for the nurse-manager to take?
1. Map out a plan of action for each problem and discuss it.
2. Begin to solve the first problem and work through the list.
3. Ask the staff member to select the problem she would like to resolve.
4. Prioritize the problems with the staff member and begin to work on them together.

2. A team leader notes increasing unrest among the staff members. Which action is best for the team leader to take?
1. Discuss the problem with a coworker.
2. Report the problem to the nurse-manager.
3. Bring the group together and discuss the team leader's perception.
4. Ignore the problem and hope the attitude won't interfere with the functioning of the floor.

3. A physician ordered a urine specimen for culture and sensitivity stat. Which approach is best for a nurse to use in delegating this task?
1. "We need a stat urine culture on the client in room 101."
2. "Please get the urine for culture for the client in room 101."
3. "A stat urine was ordered for the client in room 101. Would you get it?"
4. "We need a urine for culture stat on the client in room 101. Tell me when you send it to the lab."

1. 4. It's important for the nurse-manager and staff member to agree on which problem is a priority and work on its resolution together. Mapping out the problem without input from the staff member leaves the possibility that the staff member might not be committed to work on its resolution.
CN: Safe, effective care environment; CNS: Management of care; CL: Application

2. 3. The leader should comment to the group on the observed behavior. This is a firm approach but one that shows concern. Ignoring problems or discussing them with someone else doesn't confront the issue at hand.
CN: Safe, effective care environment; CNS: Management of care; CL: Application

3. 4. This option not only delegates the task, but also provides a checkpoint. To effectively delegate, you need to follow up on what someone else is doing. The other options don't provide for feedback, which is essential for communication and delegation.
CN: Safe, effective care environment; CNS: Management of care; CL: Application

CN: Client needs category   CNS: Client needs subcategory   TL: Cognitive level

4. A 67-year-old client asks the nurse, "Do you think it's wrong to masturbate?" Which response by the nurse is best?
 1. "How do you feel about that?"
 2. "Do you really want to do that?"
 3. "I think you're a little too old for that."
 4. "Why don't you ask your physician?"

5. A nurse is assisting a client on a clear liquid diet in selecting his menu. Which choice indicates that he needs further teaching?
 1. Gelatin dessert
 2. Milkshake
 3. Popsicle or similar frozen dessert
 4. Tea

6. Which medication should a nurse withhold from a client 6 hours before a series of pulmonary function tests (PFTs)?
 1. Antibiotics
 2. Antitussives
 3. Bronchodilators
 4. Corticosteroids

7. A client returns to a nursing unit after a bronchoscopy and is expectorating pink-tinged mucus. Which action by the nurse is most appropriate?
 1. Notify the physician as soon as possible.
 2. Take the client's vital signs, then call the physician.
 3. Auscultate the client's lung fields for possible pulmonary edema.
 4. Tell the client this is expected after the procedure, but continue to monitor the client.

4. 1. It's essential in communication to find out how the client thinks and feels. Telling the client that he's too old or asking him if he really wants to do that is biased and puts the client down. The last option tells the client the nurse isn't interested. The client might be too uncomfortable to discuss this topic with the physician.
CN: Psychosocial integrity; CNS: None; CL: Analysis

5. 2. Full-liquid diets contain milk, cereal, gruel, clear liquids, and plain frozen desserts. The clear-liquid diet contains only foods that are clear and liquid at room or body temperature, such as gelatin, fat-free broth, bouillon, popsicles or similar frozen desserts, tea, and regular or decaffeinated coffee.
CN: Physiological integrity; CNS: Basic care and comfort; CL: Analysis

6. 3. PFTs measure the volume and capacity of air. If a bronchodilator is given, it will improve the bronchial airflow and alter the test results. The other drugs would have no effect on the bronchial tree with regard to PFT results.
CN: Physiological integrity; CNS: Pharmacological and parenteral therapies; CL: Application

7. 4. Pink-tinged mucus is an expected outcome after a bronchoscopy due to irritation of the bronchial tree. The client should be told this is common, but that he'll be monitored. The physician doesn't need to be called with this finding. This symptom isn't related to pulmonary edema.
CN: Health promotion and maintenance; CNS: None; CL: Application

CN: Client needs category   CNS: Client needs subcategory   CL: Cognitive level

8. The assessment of a client on the first day after thoracotomy shows a temperature of 100° F (37.8° C); heart rate, 96 beats/minute; blood pressure, 136/86 mm Hg; and shallow respirations at 24 breaths/minute, with rhonchi at the bases. The client complains of incisional pain. Which nursing action has priority?
   1. Medicate the client for pain.
   2. Help the client get out of bed.
   3. Give ibuprofen (Motrin) as ordered to reduce the fever.
   4. Encourage the client to cough and deep-breathe.

9. Which intervention is most important to include in a nursing care plan for a client with atelectasis?
   1. Give oxygen continuously at 3 L/minute.
   2. Cough and deep-breathe every 4 hours.
   3. Use the incentive spirometer every hour.
   4. Get the client out of bed to a chair every day.

10. Two hours after submucous resection, a client's nostrils are packed and a drip pad is anchored under the nose. Which assessment alerts the nurse that the surgical site is bleeding?
   1. Frequent swallowing
   2. Dry mucous membranes
   3. Decrease in urine output
   4. Temperature elevation

11. A bedridden client develops disuse osteoporosis. Which nursing intervention is most important for this client?
   1. Turn, cough, and deep-breathe.
   2. Increase fluids to 3,000 ml daily.
   3. Promote venous return by elevating the legs.
   4. Provide active and passive range-of-motion (ROM) exercises.

You're off to a good start! Keep going!

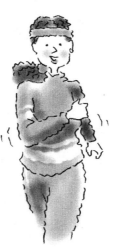

8. 1. Although all the interventions are incorporated in this client's care plan, the priority is to relieve pain and make the client comfortable. This would give the client the energy and stamina to achieve the other objectives.
CN: Physiological integrity; CNS: Basic care and comfort; CL: Application

9. 3. Incentive spirometry is used to prevent or treat atelectasis. Done every hour, it will produce deep inhalations that help open the collapsed alveoli. Oxygen use doesn't encourage deep inhalation. Coughing and deep breathing is a good intervention, but rarely results in as deep an inspiratory effort as using an incentive spirometer, and should be performed more frequently than every 4 hours. Getting the client out of bed will also help expand the lungs and stimulate deep breathing, but it's done less frequently than incentive spirometry.
CN: Safe, effective care environment; CNS: Management of care; CL: Application

10. 1. Frequent swallowing is a sign of hemorrhage in this surgery. Decreased urine output and dry mucous membranes, as well as temperature elevation, are usually signs of dehydration.
CN: Physiological integrity; CNS: Reduction of risk potential; CL: Analysis

11. 4. All the interventions listed are good for a bedridden client. However, active and passive ROM exercises provide the mechanical stresses of weight bearing that are absent and lead to disuse osteoporosis.
CN: Health promotion and maintenance; CNS: None; CL: Application

12. An elderly client on bed rest for a week after a bout of pneumonia is in a negative nitrogen balance. Which complication has highest priority?
　1. Constipation
　2. Renal calculi
　3. Muscle wasting
　4. Vitamin B_6 deficiency

12. 3. Negative nitrogen balance leads to muscle wasting. The body breaks down muscle tissue to use as energy. Renal calculi can be a complication of bed rest and demineralization of the bone but treating a negative nitrogen balance takes priority. Constipation and vitamin B_6 deficiency also need to be corrected but aren't of the highest priority.
CN: Physiological integrity; CNS: Physiological adaptation; CL: Application

13. The nurse reviews the arterial blood gas results of a client with asthma. The nurse expects the client's partial pressure of arterial oxygen (PaO_2) result to provide information on which factor?
　1. Respiratory status
　2. Degree of dyspnea
　3. Efficiency of gas exchange
　4. Effectiveness of ventilation

13. 3. The PaO_2 reflects the gas exchange ventilation and perfusion. It doesn't measure the respiratory status, degree of dyspnea, or the effectiveness of ventilation.
CN: Physiological integrity; CNS: Reduction of risk potential; CL: Application

14. The nurse prepares to administer morphine to a client with an acute myocardial infarction for which reason?
　1. To decrease cardiac output
　2. To increase preload and afterload
　3. To increase myocardial oxygen demand
　4. To decrease myocardial oxygen demand

14. 4. Morphine will calm and relax the client and decrease respiratory rate, anxiety, and stress, thus decreasing myocardial oxygen demand. It doesn't have any affect on cardiac output or preload or afterload.
CN: Physiological integrity; CNS: Pharmacological and parenteral therapies; CL: Application

15. A toddler is ordered 350 mg of amoxicillin (Augmentin) by mouth, four times per day. The pharmacy supplies a bottle of amoxicillin with a concentration of 250 mg/5 ml. How many milliliters would the nurse give for each dose? Record the answer using a whole number:
_____ml.

15. 7. The nurse would give 7 milliliters for each dose. Use the following equation:
　dose on hand/quantity on hand = dose desired/X.
　In this example, the equation is:
　250 mg/5 ml = 350 mg/X.
　X = 7 ml.
CN: Physiological integrity; CNS: Pharmacological and parenteral therapies; CL: Analysis

16. A nurse is assessing a client and notes an increase in the tactile fremitus. Which condition would the nurse suspect with this client?
　1. Atelectasis
　2. Emphysema
　3. Pneumonia
　4. Pneumothorax

16. 3. Pneumonia produces a consolidation of mucus and debris. Mucus causes the lung field to have an increase in tactile fremitus. The other diseases involve air, which would decrease tactile fremitus.
CN: Health promotion and maintenance; CNS: None; CL: Analysis

CN: Client needs category　CNS: Client needs subcategory　CL: Cognitive level

17. A client with an arm cast complains of severe pain in the affected extremity, and decreased sensation and motion are noted. Swelling in the fingers is also increased. Which intervention has priority?
    1. Elevating the arm
    2. Removing the cast
    3. Giving an analgesic
    4. Calling the physician

18. A client is hospitalized for 5 days with mononucleosis. Which assessment finding indicates a possibly serious consequence?
    1. Vomiting
    2. Dark brown urine
    3. Temperature of 101° F (38.3° C)
    4. Cervical lymphadenopathy

19. A nurse is teaching a client about lifestyle changes that need to be made after a myocardial infarction (MI). The diagnosis of *Ineffective coping* is supported when the client is observed in which action?
    1. Reading a book about meal planning
    2. Pacing the floor of his room on occasion
    3. Sitting quietly in his room for a short time
    4. Telling his family he didn't have an MI

20. A client with a history of myasthenia gravis is admitted to the emergency department with complaints of respiratory distress. The client's condition worsens and arterial blood gases are drawn. Which condition is expected?
    1. Metabolic acidosis
    2. Metabolic alkalosis
    3. Respiratory acidosis
    4. Respiratory alkalosis

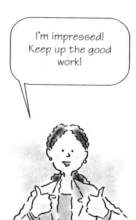

I'm impressed! Keep up the good work!

17. 4. The cast may be too tight and may need to be split or removed by the physician. Notify the physician when circulation, sensation, or motion is impaired. The arm should already be elevated. Giving analgesics wouldn't be the first step, as it may mask the signs of a serious problem.
CN: Physiological integrity; CNS: Reduction of risk potential; CL: Application

18. 2. Dark brown urine could indicate the presence of bilirubin and implicate liver involvement. The other answers are typical findings for a client with this diagnosis.
CN: Physiological integrity; CNS: Physiological adaptation; CL: Analysis

19. 4. The client is showing the defense mechanism of denial. Reading a book on meal planning is a positive intervention. Pacing the floor on occasion is a form of anxiety that's normal for the client to experience. Sitting quietly is a normal behavior. The client needs time to come to terms with his diagnosis.
CN: Psychosocial integrity; CNS: None; CL: Analysis

20. 3. The client has a restrictive lung problem because of myasthenia gravis. This is aggravated by respiratory distress. Because of the restrictive problem, the client won't be able to exhale efficiently and carbon dioxide will build up, causing respiratory acidosis. Metabolic acidosis is a metabolic condition that occurs with either accumulation of acids or excessive loss of bases in the body, such as in diarrhea or renal failure. Metabolic alkalosis occurs due to excessive acid loss or base retention, such as from vomiting. Respiratory alkalosis results from a decreased carbon dioxide level, which could occur if the patient were hyperventilating.
CN: Physiological integrity; CNS: Physiological adaptation; CL: Analysis

21. A client who had a thoracotomy is using oxygen and having an arterial blood gas (ABG) analysis. Which statement is correct to tell the client?
1. "The nurse will shave the puncture site before the test."
2. "You need to keep the oxygen mask on for the entire test."
3. "You'll be suctioned immediately before the blood is drawn."
4. "You won't be allowed to drink anything for 2 hours before the blood is drawn."

21. 2. To determine the effectiveness of oxygen therapy, ABGs are drawn with the oxygen in use. This also needs to be written on the test form. No special preparations for the test with regard to skin preparation or diet are needed. Suctioning decreases available oxygen.
CN: Physiological integrity; CNS: Basic care and comfort; CL: Application

22. Which condition causes heart failure after a myocardial infarction (MI)?
1. Increased workload of the heart
2. Increased oxygen demands of the heart
3. Inability of the heart chambers to adequately fill
4. Impairment of contractile function of the damaged myocardium

22. 4. After an MI, the injured myocardium is replaced by scar tissue. This scar tissue causes the ventricle to pump less efficiently. After an MI has resolved, oxygen and workload demands should normalize and the heart's chambers should fill adequately.
CN: Physiological integrity; CNS: Physiological adaptation; CL: Application

23. A client is admitted to the emergency department with severe epistaxis. The physician inserts posterior packing. Later, the client is anxious and says he doesn't feel he's breathing right. Which nursing action is appropriate?
1. Cut the packing strings and remove the packing.
2. Reassure the client that what he's experiencing is normal.
3. Ask the client to fully explain what he means by "right."
4. Use a flashlight and inspect the posterior oral cavity of the client.

23. 4. The nurse must assess the patency of the airway. The packing might have become dislodged. The nurse shouldn't remove the packing or give the client false reassurance. The client is too anxious to explain what he means.
CN: Physiological integrity; CNS: Reduction of risk potential; CL: Analysis

24. The nurse is teaching another nurse about pulmonary capillary wedge pressure. Which response is the most accurate regarding this pressure?
1. "It reflects systemic vascular resistance."
2. "It reflects right ventricular end pressure."
3. "It reflects right atrial presystolic pressure."
4. "It reflects left ventricular end-diastolic pressure."

24. 4. The pulmonary capillary wedge pressure is the reflection of the pressure in the left ventricle at rest, which is end diastole. Wedge pressure doesn't reflect pressures in the right side of the heart or systemic vascular resistance.
CN: Physiological integrity; CNS: Physiological adaptation; CL: Application

CN: Client needs category   CNS: Client needs subcategory   CL: Cognitive level

25. The nurse is teaching a student nurse about the purpose of diaphragmatic breathing exercises for a client with chronic obstructive pulmonary disease (COPD). Which statement by the nurse is correct?
1. "It dilates the bronchioles."
2. "It decreases vital capacity."
3. "It increases residual volume."
4. "It decreases alveolar ventilation."

26. A client with chronic obstructive pulmonary disease (COPD) is being discharged from the hospital. The nurse provided teaching on medications, diet, and exercise. Which statement by the client indicates more teaching is needed?
1. "I'll eat six small meals a day."
2. "I'll get a flu shot every winter."
3. "I'll walk every morning before breakfast."
4. "I'll call my physician if I get cold symptoms."

27. The nurse is caring for a client showing symptoms of bronchial obstruction. Which assessment finding would the nurse expect to find?
1. Hacking cough
2. Diminished breath sounds
3. Production of rust-colored sputum
4. Decreased use of accessory muscles

28. A client has just started treatment with Rifampin for tuberculosis. Which statement indicates the client has a good understanding of his medication?
1. "I won't go to family gatherings for 6 months."
2. "My urine will look orange because of the medication."
3. "Now I don't need to cover my mouth or nose when I sneeze or cough."
4. "I told my wife to throw away all the spoons and forks before I come home."

25. 1. In COPD, the bronchioles constrict during exhalation due to pressure changes in the lungs. Diaphragmatic breathing exercises keep the bronchioles open during exhalation. These exercises aren't performed for the other reasons stated.
CN: Physiological integrity; CNS: Reduction of risk potential; CL: Application

26. 3. The worst time of the day for a client with COPD is morning. Exercise is important, but should be done later in the day. All other choices are appropriate for the client with COPD.
CN: Physiological integrity; CNS: Basic care and comfort; CL: Application

27. 2. Bronchial obstruction means no passage of air through the bronchi, so diminished or no breath sounds would be heard. A hacking cough is often associated with upper respiratory tract infection and dryness in the upper airways. Rust-colored sputum is a sign of pneumococcal pneumonia. There would be increased use of accessory muscles.
CN: Physiological integrity; CNS: Physiological adaptation; CL: Application

28. 2. Rifampin discolors body fluids, such as urine and tears. The client can go to family functions and eat with normal utensils. The client should cover his mouth and nose when coughing and sneezing until he has been on the medication at least 2 weeks.
CN: Physiological integrity; CNS: Pharmacological and parenteral therapies; CL: Application

29. Before feeding a client with Parkinson's disease, which nursing action is most important?
    1. Sit the client upright.
    2. Have suction available.
    3. Order a clear liquid diet.
    4. Have a speech therapist evaluate the client.

30. The nurse is caring for a pregnant client with cardiovascular disease. Which treatment would the nurse expect for this client?
    1. Rest
    2. Hospitalization
    3. Therapeutic abortion
    4. Continuous cardiac monitoring

31. Which assessment finding most likely indicates a urinary tract infection (UTI) in a 5-year-old child?
    1. Incontinence
    2. Lack of thirst
    3. Concentrated urine
    4. Subnormal temperature

32. During a home health visit, a nurse assesses a client's medication and notes the client has two prescriptions for fluid retention. One prescription reads "Lasix, 40 mg, one tablet daily." The next prescription reads "Furosemide, 40 mg, one tablet daily." Which instruction is given to the client?
    1. Take both medications as ordered.
    2. Lasix and furosemide are the same drug.
    3. Use Lasix one day and furosemide the next day.
    4. Throw away one of the drugs to avoid confusing the client.

29. 4. A speech therapist can evaluate the client's swallowing and make recommendations before the client is fed. Aspiration due to involuntary movement is common. Sitting the client upright and having suction available are helpful when feeding the client, but evaluation of the client's swallowing ability should come first. Clear liquids may be too difficult for the client; semisoft foods may be easier to swallow.
CN: Physiological integrity; CNS: Reduction of risk potential; CL: Analysis

30. 1. The goal of antepartum management is to prevent complications and minimize the strain on the client. This is done with rest. Hospitalization may be required in older women or those with previous decompensation. Therapeutic abortion is considered in severe dysfunction, especially in the first trimester. Continuous cardiac monitoring isn't necessary.
CN: Physiological integrity; CNS: Reduction of risk potential; CL: Application

31. 1. Incontinence in a toilet-trained child is associated with UTI. Lack of thirst wouldn't be expected in a child with UTI. Concentrated urine is a sign of dehydration. Subnormal temperature isn't a sign of UTI.
CN: Health promotion and maintenance; CNS: None; CL: Application

32. 2. Using generic names for medications is common, especially for home health clients. It's the responsibility of the nurse to teach the client both brand and generic names of drugs. Setting up medications in a medication tray, using only one pharmacy to dispense medications, and using all medications until the bottle is emptied will reduce medication errors.
CN: Physiological integrity; CNS: Pharmacological and parenteral therapies; CL: Analysis

CN: Client needs category   CNS: Client needs subcategory   CL: Cognitive level

33. A school nurse is called to assess a preadolescent Vietnamese girl attending a new school. A teacher tells the nurse the student sits in the back of the class and won't speak when spoken to, although her parents confirmed the student speaks English. Which assessment finding is most likely?
1. The student is experiencing cultural shock.
2. The student is developing a peer support system.
3. The student is going through a socialization period.
4. The student is becoming acculturated to the new school.

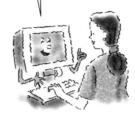

You're doing sensationally! You really know your stuff!

33. 1. Cultural shock is a feeling of helplessness, discomfort, and a state of disorientation when an outsider attempts to comprehend or adapt to a new cultural situation. Peer groups usually develop based on the background, interests, and capabilities of its members. Developing peer cultures is part of the socialization process. Acculturation occurs when there's a blending of cultural or ethnic backgrounds. This process takes time to develop.
CN: Health promotion and maintenance; CNS: None; CL: Application

34. A school nurse is screening for hearing and vision with a group of 11- to 13-year-old students. Which technique is used to communicate effectively with this age group?
1. Give undivided attention to each student.
2. Have the parents present during the screening.
3. Have several adolescents listen to each other's health histories.
4. Use puppets or dolls to show how the screening is going to take place.

34. 1. Give undivided attention to communicate effectively with adolescents. Respect their privacy. The presence of parents and use of puppets or dolls can be used to effectively communicate with younger children.
CN: Health promotion and maintenance; CNS: None; CL: Application

35. A nurse practitioner at a rural health clinic is screening an 18-month-old infant for developmental problems. Which developmental screening test is the most appropriate?
1. Goodenough-Harris Draw-a-Person Test
2. Denver Developmental Screening Test (DDST)
3. McCarthy Scales of Children's Abilities (MSCA)
4. Preschool readiness screening scales

35. 2. The DDST is applicable for children from birth through age 6. The Goodenough-Harris Draw-a-Person Test is used to assess intellectual ability in children ages 3 to 10. The MSCA is a developmental tool for children ages 2½ to 8½. Preschool readiness screening scales are designed for screening 5-year-old children for readiness for school.
CN: Health promotion and maintenance; CNS: None; CL: Application

36. In preparing an educational intervention for college students, a nurse understands that drinking alcoholic beverages is often used to relieve which condition?
1. Fatigue
2. Anxiety
3. Headache
4. Stomach pain

36. 2. Drinking alcoholic beverages is commonly thought to alleviate anxiety. These beverages aren't commonly used to relieve fatigue, headache, or stomach pain.
CN: Psychosocial integrity; CNS: None; CL: Application

37. An educational forum about relaxation techniques is provided for college students preparing for their final exams. Which relaxation technique is most effective to counteract anxiety?
  1. Meditation
  2. Music therapy
  3. Dance therapy
  4. Reality orientation

38. The parents of a 9-year-old child diagnosed with oppositional defiant disorder (ODD) are discussing treatment options with the nurse. Which action would the nurse expect to have the most positive impact on managing the child's behavior?
  1. Daily administration of methylphenidate hydrochloride (Ritalin)
  2. Providing praise to the child for positive behaviors
  3. Including the child in group therapy with other children diagnosed with ODD
  4. Assigning several household chores to the child for weekly completion

39. A 40-year-old female client is admitted to a women's shelter after being raped by her estranged husband. The client describes the traumatic event. Which response by the nurse is best?
  1. Change the subject to prevent the client from crying.
  2. Listen attentively while the client describes the event.
  3. Arrange for the client to tell her story in group therapy.
  4. Medicate the client with a tranquilizer to prevent hysteria.

40. A nurse is assessing a client with manic-depressive disorder. The client tells the nurse his family physician prescribed lithium. Which symptom indicates the client is developing lithium toxicity?
  1. Lethargy
  2. Hypertension
  3. Hyperexcitability
  4. Low urine output

37. 1. Meditation is a relaxation therapy used to counteract anxiety related to stress-inducing internal and external stimuli. Music therapy, dance therapy, and reality orientation are used as adjuncts to psychiatric care.
CN: Psychosocial integrity; CNS: None; CL: Application

38. 2. Children with ODD consistently display negativity, defiance to authority, and hostility. ODD is best managed with consistent parenting and the establishment of a warm, positive home environment. Medication therapies aren't typically used for children with ODD. Methylphenidate is commonly used to manage attention deficit disorder. The focus of treatment for ODD is on the family unit, not on other children with similar problems. The child should be asked to participate in chores, but the parents need to be aware that overwhelming tasks may cause frustration and more defiance.
CN: Psychosocial integrity; CNS: None; CL: Analysis

39. 2. Retelling the event is part of the healing process. Giving medication and changing the subject don't allow the client to integrate the experience into her life. Group therapy may be helpful, but the best nursing response is to listen and convey empathy.
CN: Psychosocial integrity; CNS: None; CL: Application

40. 1. Nausea, vomiting, diarrhea, thirst, polyuria, lethargy, slurred speech, hypotension, muscle weakness, and fine hand tremors are signs of lithium toxicity.
CN: Physiological integrity; CNS: Pharmacological and parenteral therapies; CL: Application

CN: Client needs category   CNS: Client needs subcategory   CL: Cognitive level

41. Which nursing intervention is used during assessment of a pediatric client?
1. Ask the parents to leave the room during health assessment.
2. Position the client on an examination table or bed at all times.
3. Organize the health assessment in the same way for every infant or child.
4. Identify the source (child, parent, caregiver, guardian) and indicate the reliability of the information obtained.

42. Which nursing intervention is used during assessment of an elderly client?
1. Ask the client to change positions quickly.
2. Keep the room temperature cool during health assessment.
3. Speak loudly and quickly to facilitate understanding of directions.
4. Change the height of the examination table or modify the client's position.

43. Which nursing diagnosis is appropriate for a client with chronic obstructive pulmonary disease who is anxious, dyspneic, and hypoxic?
1. *Ineffective breathing pattern related to anxiety*
2. *Risk for aspiration related to absence of protective mechanisms*
3. *Impaired gas exchange related to altered oxygen-carrying capacity of the blood*
4. *Ineffective airway clearance related to presence of tracheobronchial obstruction or secretions*

44. Which statement is a wellness nursing diagnosis?
1. *Readiness for enhanced spiritual well-being*
2. *Risk for activity intolerance related to prolonged bed rest*
3. *Bathing self-care deficit related to fatigue and muscular weakness*
4. *Constipation related to decreased activity and fluid intake as manifested by hard, formed stool every 3 days*

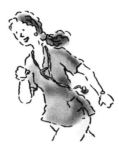

More than halfway home! Excellent!

41. 4. Document the source of information obtained for the nursing assessment of a child. Separation from the parent may cause anxiety and increase the child's fear and distrust. Depending on the child's age, parents may help position and hold the child, facilitating assessment. Organization of the assessment is changed to accommodate the individual child's age and development.
CN: Health promotion and maintenance; CNS: None; CL: Application

42. 4. You may need to change the height of the examination table or use a different position when assessing an elderly client. Physiologically, an older client is prone to falls and dizziness due to decreased ability to respond to sudden movements and position changes. The room temperature should be warm because older clients become hypothermic easily. Speak in a slow, normal tone of voice to facilitate communication.
CN: Health promotion and maintenance; CNS: None; CL: Application

43. 3. The correct nursing diagnosis for this client is based on the impaired oxygenation at the cellular level. The first option applies to a client whose inhalation or exhalation pattern doesn't enable adequate pulmonary inflation or emptying. The second option applies if the client is at risk for aspirating gastric or pharyngeal secretions, food, or fluids into the tracheobronchial passages. The last option is appropriate for a client who's unable to clear secretions or obstructions from the respiratory tract.
CN: Safe, effective care environment; CNS: Management of care; CL: Application

44. 1. Wellness diagnoses are one-part statements containing the label only and begin with "*Readiness for enhanced,*" followed by the higher level of wellness desired for the individual or group. The second option is a "risk for" nursing diagnosis. The third option describes a suspected problem for which additional data are needed for confirmation. The last option describes a manifested health problem validated by identifiable major defining characteristics.
CN: Safe, effective care environment; CNS: Management of care; CL: Application

45. A nurse observes that a client with a below-the-knee amputation on the third post-operative day refuses to look at the stump and changes the subject when the nurse attempts to discuss its care. Which nursing diagnosis should the nurse use to address this situation?
1. *Hopelessness*
2. *Impaired physical mobility*
3. *Disturbed body image*
4. *Powerlessness*

45. 3. Refusing to look at the stump is a characteristic of *Disturbed body image.* Other defining characteristics include having a missing body part, hiding a body part, and negative feelings about one's body. The other nursing diagnoses may also be appropriate for this client, but the data presented best reflects *Disturbed body image. Hopelessness* occurs when a person sees limited or no alternatives and is unable to mobilize energy to act. *Impaired physical mobility* may also occur in the client following an amputation, but the data presented doesn't support this diagnosis. With *Power-lessness,* the client doesn't believe his actions will have an effect. Again, the data presented doesn't support this diagnosis.
CN: Safe, effective care environment; CNS: Management of care; CL: Analysis

46. An intake nurse at a mental health facility is admitting a client with psychosis. Which assessment technique is most valuable to use when planning this client's care?
1. Rorschach test
2. Interview with the client
3. Mental Status Examination (MSE)
4. Review old records of the client

46. 3. The MSE is a basis for planning care with a mental health client, especially one who's psychotic. The Rorschach test is used for depression. An interview with a client with psychosis would be unreliable. Review of old records won't assess the current state on which interventions are planned.
CN: Psychosocial integrity; CNS: None; CL: Application

47. Which is a sign that a client with a new diagnosis of breast cancer is having difficulty coping?
1. The client cries when discussing her diagnosis.
2. The client asks questions about treatment.
3. The client is concerned about missing work during chemotherapy.
4. The client changes the topic when treatment is discussed.

47. 4. By changing the topic when breast cancer treatment is discussed, the client may be denying her condition and having difficulty coping. It is normal to cry, ask questions, and be concerned about missing work when discussing a diagnosis such as breast cancer.
CN: Psychosocial integrity; CNS: None; CL: Application

48. Which patient outcome or goal should a nurse identify for a client with the nursing diagnosis *Risk for disuse syndrome?*
1. The client will be free of musculoskeletal complications.
2. The client will experience shorter periods of immobility and inactivity.
3. The nurse will stress the importance of maintaining adequate fluid intake.
4. The nurse will provide holistic care by collaborating with the health care team.

48. 2. This is an appropriate outcome for a client with this nursing diagnosis. Disuse syndrome, a result of prolonged or unavoidable immobility or inactivity, can be prevented. Musculoskeletal complications indicate actual disuse or complications of immobility. Stressing the importance of adequate fluid intake and providing holistic care describe nursing goals, not patient outcomes.
CN: Safe, effective care environment; CNS: Management of care; CL: Application

CN: Client needs category   CNS: Client needs subcategory   CL: Cognitive level

49. A 42-year-old client who underwent a right modified mastectomy with insertion of a Hemovac drain will be hospitalized overnight because of minor complications. Which goal statement should the nurse include in the plan of care?
   1. Teach proper care of the incision site and drain by October 12.
   2. The client will know how to care for the incision site and drain by October 12.
   3. The client will show the proper care of the incision site and drain by October 12.
   4. The client will care for the incision site and contend with psychological loss by October 12.

50. Which expected outcome or goal should a nurse identify for a client with the nursing diagnosis *Risk for injury related to lack of awareness of environmental hazards?*
   1. Encourage the client to discuss safety rules with children.
   2. Help the client learn safety precautions to take in the home.
   3. The client will eliminate safety hazards in his surroundings.
   4. The client will contact community resources for more information.

51. What is the best action by a nurse when talking with a client diagnosed with prostate cancer who is tearful and having difficulty talking about his concerns?
   1. Ask if he would like to speak with a chaplain.
   2. Tell the client that she will be back once he has stopped crying.
   3. Sit and ask him if he would like to talk about his concerns.
   4. Tell the client that she knows how he is feeling.

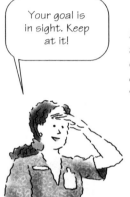

Your goal is in sight. Keep at it!

49. 3. This statement contains a specific measurable verb, clearly identifies the client behavior, and includes a date. Option 1 is a nursing goal as written, not a client-centered goal. The client goal of option 2 isn't measurable as stated. Option 4 includes two goals that need to be addressed separately under the appropriate nursing diagnosis and it contains nonmeasurable verbs.
CN: Physiological integrity; CNS: Basic care and comfort; CL: Application

50. 3. This goal is appropriate and measurable as written and focuses on the client. The other options are nursing interventions as written.
CN: Safe, effective care environment; CNS: Management of care; CL: Application

51. 3. By sitting down, the nurse shows the client that he is important. Asking if he would like to talk about his concerns lets the client know that the nurse cares about him and wants to help. Calling a chaplain is appropriate after the nurse has assessed the situation and the client has verbalized his concerns. Telling the client that she will return after he stops crying does not show concern for his feelings and does not encourage verbalization. Telling the client that she understands how he feels doesn't help him verbalize his feelings.
CN: Psychosocial integrity; CNS: None; CL: Application

52. A client with heart failure is given furosemide (Lasix) 40 mg I.V. daily. The morning serum potassium level is 2.8 mEq/L. Which nursing action is the most appropriate?
1. Question the physician about the dosage.
2. Give 20 mg of the ordered dose and recheck the laboratory test results.
3. Notify the physician, repeat the potassium as ordered, then give the furosemide.
4. Give the furosemide and get an order for sodium polystyrene sulfonate.

52. 3. Furosemide is a diuretic. As water is lost, so is potassium. Diuresis is a treatment for heart failure. Notifying the physician of the low potassium level and getting an order for potassium chloride is the appropriate action before giving the furosemide. Furosemide, 40 mg, is an appropriate dose for the treatment of heart failure. The nurse shouldn't give half the dose without an order. Giving furosemide and sodium polystyrene sulfonate together would further lower the potassium level.
CN: Physiological integrity; CNS: Pharmacological and parenteral therapies; CL: Application

53. Which client is at greatest risk for developing respiratory alkalosis?
1. A client in labor
2. A client with diabetes
3. A client with renal failure
4. An immediate postoperative client

53. 1. A client's respirations at certain stages of labor increase in volume, causing the $Paco_2$ to decrease, increasing the pH. Diabetes often causes a metabolic imbalance, resulting in metabolic acidosis. In renal failure, the inability of the kidneys to eliminate wastes increases the risk of developing metabolic acidosis. The respirations of a postoperative client are usually shallow after anesthesia and, because of pain, often cause respiratory acidosis.
CN: Physiological integrity; CNS: Physiological adaptation; CL: Analysis

54. Which condition indicates to a nurse that a sterile field has been contaminated?
1. Sterile objects are held above the waist of the nurse.
2. Sterile packages are opened with the first edge away from the nurse.
3. The outer inch of the sterile towel hangs over the side of the table.
4. Wetness on the sterile cloth on top of the nonsterile table has been noted.

54. 4. Moisture outside the sterile package and field contaminates it because fluid can be wicked into the sterile field. Bacteria tend to settle, so there's less contamination above waist level and away from the nurse. The outer inch of the drape is considered contaminated but doesn't indicate that the sterile field itself has been contaminated.
CN: Safe, effective care environment; CNS: Safety and infection control; CL: Application

55. Which intervention should a nurse perform for a client with respiratory alkalosis?
1. Have the client breathe into a paper bag.
2. Give one ampule of bicarbonate as ordered.
3. Give oxygen at 3 L/minute through a nasal cannula.
4. Reposition the client in a high Fowler's position.

55. 1. By breathing into a paper bag, the client will rebreathe some of his own exhaled carbon dioxide and increase the carbon dioxide in his blood, which will correct his respiratory alkalosis. Giving one ampule of bicarbonate will worsen the alkalosis. Giving oxygen won't increase the carbon dioxide to correct the imbalance. Repositioning the client won't help him retain carbon dioxide.
CN: Physiological integrity; CNS: Physiological adaptation; CL: Analysis

CN: Client needs category   CNS: Client needs subcategory   CL: Cognitive level

56. The nurse is reviewing the laboratory results from a female diabetic client admitted to the acute care facility with dehydration. Which laboratory result is consistent with a diagnosis of dehydration?
1. Serum hematocrit of 40%
2. Urine dipstick specific gravity of 1.035
3. Serum creatinine level of 0.8 mg/dl
4. HbA$_{1c}$ level of 4%

56. 2. Urine specific gravity reflects the ability of the kidneys to concentrate urine. Normal urine specific gravity is 1.005 to 1.030. A higher urine specific gravity indicates that the urine is more concentrated, and this is consistent with dehydration. The normal hematocrit range for a female client is 36% to 48%, so this value is within normal limits. Dehydration would cause an increase in hematocrit. Serum creatinine is used to assess kidney function. The normal range for women is 0.6 to 0.9 mg/dl. HbA$_{1c}$ is used to monitor diabetes treatment and evaluate the average blood glucose over a period of months. The normal range for HbA$_{1c}$ is 4% to 6.7%.
CN: Physiological integrity; CNS: Physiological adaptation; CL: Analysis

57. A client admitted with hypoparathyroidism is being monitored for hypocalcemia. Which finding would the nurse observe with hypocalcemia?
1. Battle's sign
2. Brudzinski's sign
3. Chvostek's sign
4. Homans' sign

57. 3. Hypocalcemia can cause Chvostek's sign, abnormal facial muscle and nerve spasms elicited when the facial nerve is tapped. Battle's sign is bruising over the temporal bone in the presence of a basilar skull fracture. Brudzinski's sign is the flexion of the hips and knees in response to flexion of the head and neck toward the chest, indicating meningeal irritation. A positive Homans' sign indicates deep vein thrombosis.
CN: Physiological integrity; CNS: Reduction of risk potential; CL: Application

58. A client is complaining of pain 1 day after a colostomy. The nurse gives morphine I.M. and, 30 minutes later, finds the respiratory rate at 8 breaths/minute, with the nasal cannula on the floor. Arterial blood gas (ABG) results are pH, 7.23; Pao$_2$, 58 mm Hg; Paco$_2$, 61 mm Hg; HCO$_3^-$, 24 mEq/L. Which group of factors contributes most to this client's ABG results?
1. Colostomy, pain, and morphine
2. Morphine, the nasal cannula on the floor, and the colostomy
3. Morphine, respiratory rate of 8 breaths/minute, and the nasal cannula on the floor
4. Pain, respiratory rate of 8 breaths/minute, and the nasal cannula on the floor

58. 3. This client has respiratory acidosis. Opioids can suppress respirations, causing retention of carbon dioxide. A Pao$_2$ of 58 mm Hg indicates hypoxemia, which is caused by the removal of the client's supplementary oxygen and the decreased respiratory rate. Pain increases—not decreases—the respiratory rate, which causes a decrease in Paco$_2$. Colostomy drainage doesn't start until 2 to 3 days postoperatively, and this drainage would contribute to metabolic alkalosis.
CN: Physiological integrity; CNS: Physiological adaptation; CL: Analysis

59. Which arterial blood gas (ABG) results should a nurse expect to see in a client with emphysema?
1. pH, 7.52; $Paco_2$, 18 mm Hg; HCO_3^-, 22 mEq/L
2. pH, 7.50; $Paco_2$, 38 mm Hg; HCO_3^-, 38 mEq/L
3. pH, 7.30; $Paco_2$, 52 mm Hg; HCO_3^-, 30 mEq/L
4. pH, 7.30; $Paco_2$, 40 mm Hg; HCO_3^-, 18 mEq/L

60. Which factor does a nurse identify as a major cause of metabolic alkalosis in a client who had a colon resection?
1. Hyperventilation
2. Pain management
3. Nasogastric suction
4. I.V. therapy

61. Which nursing action should be included in the plan of care to prevent an increase in intracranial pressure (ICP) in a comatose client with a closed head injury?
1. Suction the airway every hour to maintain patency.
2. Elevate the head of the bed 20 degrees.
3. Place in a supine position with the head turned to the side.
4. Provide environmental stimulation.

62. After making the bed of a client with dementia, which action has priority?
1. Put the bed in the lowest position.
2. Put the call button within the client's reach.
3. Put the top side rails in the upright position.
4. Put soiled linen in a hamper or biohazard bag.

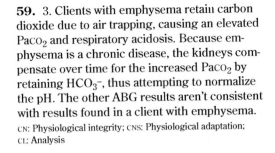

Only 15 more to go!

59. 3. Clients with emphysema retain carbon dioxide due to air trapping, causing an elevated $Paco_2$ and respiratory acidosis. Because emphysema is a chronic disease, the kidneys compensate over time for the increased $Paco_2$ by retaining HCO_3^-, thus attempting to normalize the pH. The other ABG results aren't consistent with results found in a client with emphysema.
CN: Physiological integrity; CNS: Physiological adaptation; CL: Analysis

60. 3. Removing acidic gastric secretions from the stomach is a metabolic cause of alkalinization of the blood pH. Hyperventilation decreases carbon dioxide and increases the pH, causing respiratory alkalosis. Pain management may further decrease the respiratory rate. Most I.V. fluids don't influence pH.
CN: Physiological integrity; CNS: Physiological adaptation; CL: Analysis

61. 2. The head of the bed should be elevated between 15 to 30 degrees to promote venous drainage. Suctioning the airway may increase ICP and should only be performed when needed. Turning the head to the side may cause jugular venous compression and an elevation in ICP. Environmental stimulation should be minimized to reduce any rise in ICP.
CN: Physiological integrity; CNS: Reduction in risk potential; CL: Application

62. 1. To reduce the risk of injury due to falls, the bed should be placed in the lowest position. The call button should be in reach of the client, but the immediate safety of the client comes first. All four side rails should be up to prevent accidental falls and to remind clients to stay in bed. Soiled linens should be placed in a hamper or biohazard bag, but client safety is a priority.
CN: Safe, effective care environment; CNS: Management of care; CL: Application

63. After emptying urine from the bedpan of a client whose urinary output is being monitored, which step should a nurse do next?

1. Wash hands thoroughly.
2. Apply a clean pair of gloves.
3. Report the amount of urine to the nurse in charge right away.
4. Document the amount and characteristics of urine in the chart.

63. 1. After any procedure is completed, the nurse must wash her hands to prevent transmission of microorganisms. The application of gloves is only necessary if the nurse must attend to another item of personal care before documenting urinary output; even so, hands should be washed first. Crucial information is reported to the charge nurse, not routine intake and output. Documentation should take place, but following the handwashing.

CN: Safe, effective care environment; CNS: Safety and infection control; CL: Application

64. Which client should a nurse place in an orthopneic position?

1. A client with edema of the lower legs and ankles
2. A client with a pressure ulcer on the coccyx and buttocks
3. An immobilized client with calf tenderness due to a thrombus
4. An elderly client with difficulty breathing

64. 4. The orthopneic position, which is appropriate for a client with breathing difficulty, is a sitting position with the arms leaning on a bedside table. Sitting with the legs elevated to decrease edema is appropriate for clients with ankle and lower leg swelling. A client with a pressure ulcer will need to be positioned on his side and turned every 2 hours. Fowler's or semi-Fowler's positions are most appropriate for a client on complete bed rest.

CN: Physiological integrity; CNS: Physiological adaptation; CL: Application

65. A client preparing to transfer from the bed to a wheelchair complains of feeling light-headed and dizzy as he rises from a supine to a sitting position. Which action should the nurse take next?

1. Lift the client quickly into the wheelchair.
2. Return the client to the supine position and apply a safety vest.
3. Ask the client to dangle his legs at the bedside while leaving the room for a few seconds to get assistance.
4. Have the client sit at the side of the bed for a few minutes while supporting his back and shoulders.

65. 4. A quick change in position will decrease the blood pressure, causing momentary light-headedness and dizziness. An additional change in position may further reduce the client's blood pressure to a level that may require emergency assistance. This can be avoided by waiting with the client in the sitting position until the blood pressure stabilizes. A safety vest isn't necessary. Leaving the room may put the client in danger if the blood pressure decreases further and the client needs emergency assistance. If the client continues to complain of dizziness and light-headedness, then return the client to bed.

CN: Physiological integrity; CNS: Reduction of risk potential; CL: Application

66. Which nursing action is the most effective infection control measure for preventing the transmission of microorganisms?

1. Change a client's bed linen daily.
2. Wash hands before and after client contact.
3. Wear sterile gloves when touching a client's skin.
4. Wear a mask when in direct contact with infected clients.

67. The nurse is teaching a student nurse about standard precautions. Which action by the student nurse indicates that the teaching has been effective?

1. Wear eye goggles while giving a complete bed bath.
2. Recap a needle used for an injection before disposal.
3. Dispose of blood-contaminated materials in a biohazard container.
4. Use alcohol to decontaminate blood-contaminated steel instruments.

68. A team leader would instruct team members to wear a mask and protective eyewear or a face shield in which situation?

1. When strong odors are emitted from an infected wound
2. When the client has an oral temperature greater than 101° F (38.3° C)
3. If needles or other sharp instruments are to be used in the procedure
4. During a procedure where splashing of blood or body fluid is anticipated

69. A nurse is caring for a client on neutropenic precautions. At which time should the nurse remove the barrier protection when leaving the room?

1. Within the client's room, just inside the doorway
2. Out of the client's room, just outside the doorway
3. In the hallway, a significant distance from the client's room
4. At the bedside, immediately after completing work with the client

66. 2. Typically, the transmission of microorganisms occurs when health care personnel don't wash their hands before and after touching a client or contaminated objects. A daily linen change isn't the most effective method of controlling infection. Sterile gloves and a mask aren't needed during routine client care.
CN: Safe, effective care environment; CNS: Safety and infection control; CL: Application

67. 3. Blood-contaminated materials are disposed of in a biohazard container. Recapping needles puts the health care provider at risk for sticking himself. Standard precautions needn't be observed during a bath because of the low risk for exposure to blood. Blood-contaminated steel instruments are decontaminated in an autoclave.
CN: Safe, effective care environment; CNS: Safety and infection control; CL: Application

68. 4. Wearing eye goggles or face shields prevents blood or body-fluid splashes into the eyes. Odors don't transmit microorganisms. A client with a fever won't transmit microorganisms into the eyes any more frequently than a client without a fever. The use of needles or other sharp instruments doesn't mandate eye protection.
CN: Safe, effective environment; CNS: Management of care; CL: Application

69. 2. Disposing of gowns and gloves just outside the doorway provides sufficient distance from the client for all but airborne microorganisms. The client is protected from infection by airborne pathogens by keeping the door shut as much as possible to decrease the chance of exposure. Disposal of barriers at the bedside or inside the door negates the effectiveness of wearing barriers in the first place. It's unnecessary to wear the barriers away from the doorway as the door should remain closed.
CN: Safe, effective care environment; CNS: Safety and infection control; CL: Application

CN: Client needs category CNS: Client needs subcategory CL: Cognitive level

70. Which timeframe is most appropriate for completing client teaching for a client undergoing an open cholecystectomy?
1. The day of discharge
2. A few weeks before the surgery
3. The first 12 hours after surgery
4. Before discharge, 1 to 2 days after the surgery

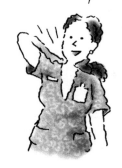

Pat yourself on the back. Only five more to go.

71. Which technique is appropriate for promoting proper breathing in a client experiencing pain or anxiety?
1. Rapid, light respirations
2. Rapid, deep respirations
3. In through the mouth and out through the nose
4. In through the nose and out through the mouth

72. The nurse is assessing a client who was admitted with a pressure ulcer. The nurse determines that the ulcer is at stage II. Which graphic represents stage II of a pressure ulcer?

1.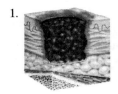
2.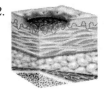
3.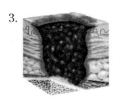
4.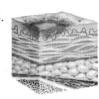

70. 4. Pain levels should have sufficiently subsided 1 to 2 days after the surgical procedure, allowing the client to concentrate on the information. The day of discharge is too late, because it doesn't give the client time to ask questions or practice procedures (such as syringe preparation) that may be necessary. Also, the individual may be anxious about returning home, which may interfere with learning. A few weeks before surgery is generally too early to retain information, and teaching within the first 12 hours after surgery isn't likely to produce retention of information, either.
CN: Physiological integrity; CNS: Physiological adaptation; CL: Application

71. 4. Air inhaled through the nose is warmed, humidified, and filtered for large particles with the nasal hairs, conditioning the air for delivery to the lungs. Exhaling through the mouth after inhaling through the nose requires some concentration and provides a focus to distract a client experiencing pain and anxiety. This method is used to control respiratory rates when clients are anxious or in pain and optimizes air exchange. Rapid, light, or deep respirations cause the client to lose oxygen exchange time while continuing to blow off carbon dioxide. This leads to hypoxemia and respiratory alkalosis.
CN: Physiological integrity; CNS: Physiological adaptation; CL; Application

72. 2. Stage II is marked by partial-thickness skin loss that involves the epidermis, dermis, or both, with an abrasion, blister, or shallow crater. The first graphic is stage III, which is a full-thickness wound that appears like a deep crater. The third graphic is of stage IV, which involves all thicknesses and involves the muscle, bone, and supporting structures. The fourth graphic is of stage I, which is a reddened area with intact skin or, in those with dark skin, there may be warmth, edema, discoloration, induration, or hardness.
CN: Physiological integrity; CNS: Physiological adaptation; CL: Analysis

73. A 46-year-old single female client was concerned about her 15-year-old son's behavior. He suddenly decided his mother shouldn't date or have men in the house. He told his mother he was the "man of the house." Which disturbance was occurring in the internal dynamics of the family?

1. Age-appropriate behavior is occurring.
2. The son is powerful in the family system.
3. The son is trying to establish a role reversal.
4. It's culturally acceptable to be the man of the house at age 15.

73. 3. Role reversal occurs when the patterns of expected behavior aren't appropriate to age and ability. Males ages 13 to 17 are developing their identities, and separation from parents becomes necessary for individuation to occur. Males have a better understanding of their roles in relationships and families if they're raised around strong male role models. In healthy families, power is shared appropriate to age until the children are independent.

CN: Psychosocial integrity; CNS: None; CL: Analysis

74. A nurse is reviewing the causes of gastroesophageal reflux disease (GERD) with a client. What area of the GI tract should the nurse identify as the cause of reduced pressure associated with GERD?

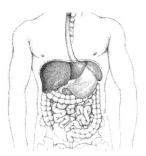

74. Normally, there is enough pressure around the lower esophageal sphincter (LES) to close it. Reflux occurs when LES pressure is deficient or when pressure in the stomach exceeds LES pressure.

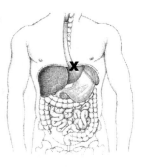

CN: Health promotion and maintenance; CNS: None; CL: Application

75. A nurse is preparing a client with a tracheostomy for discharge. Which statements by the client indicate that he understands the teaching regarding his tracheostomy care?

1. "I will need to cover the opening when I shower."
2. "I can swim as long as I keep my head above water."
3. "I will need to wash my hands after caring for my tracheostomy."
4. "I will need to take antibiotics to prevent infections."

75. 1. The opening will require protection when bathing. Swimming isn't recommended; drowning can occur even if the client's head isn't submerged. It's necessary to wash hands before and after caring for the tracheostomy. Prophylactic antibiotics aren't required for the client with a tracheostomy.

CN: Safe, effective care environment; CNS: Safety and infection control; CL: Application

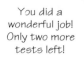

You did a wonderful job! Only two more tests left!

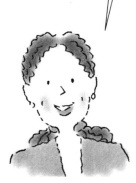

CN: Client needs category   CNS: Client needs subcategory   CL: Cognitive level

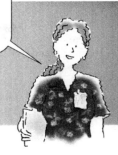

COMPREHENSIVE
Test 5

1. Which information about vital signs should a nurse report to the physician?
1. Blood pressure of 120/72 mm Hg in a healthy man
2. Pulse of 110 beats/minute on awakening in the morning
3. Blood pressure of 110/68 mm Hg in a healthy woman
4. Pulse of 120 beats/minute after 30 minutes of aerobic exercise

2. Immediately after a client's cardiac catheterization via the femoral artery, the client is being assessed by the nurse. Which assessment finding would the nurse report immediately to the physician?
1. Apical pulse of 98 beats/minute
2. Dressing with dime-sized red drainage
3. Absence of dorsalis pedis pulse
4. Blood pressure of 105/70 mm Hg

3. A nurse is preparing to bathe a client who's hospitalized for emphysema. Which nursing intervention is correct?
1. Remove the oxygen and proceed with the bath.
2. Increase the flow of oxygen to 6 L/minute by nasal cannula.
3. Keep the head of the bed slightly elevated during the procedure.
4. Lower the head of the bed and roll the client to his left side to increase oxygenation.

1. 2. The normal range for a pulse is 60 to 100 beats/minute and, in the morning, the rate is at its lowest. Blood pressures of 120/72 mm Hg for a healthy man and 110/68 mm Hg for a healthy woman are normal. Aerobic exercise increases the heart rate over the normal range of 60 to 100 beats/minute. The formula for maximum aerobic heart rate is: 210 − age × 80%. A person shouldn't go over the maximum heart rate during aerobic exercise.
CN: Physiological integrity; CNS: Physiological adaptation; CL: Analysis

2. 3. The dorsalis pedis is the pulse used to determine peripheral circulation to the lower extremities after a cardiac catheterization. Absence of this pulse should be reported immediately to the physician. An apical pulse of 98 beats/minute and a blood pressure of 105/70 mm Hg are within the normal range. A dressing with dime-sized, red drainage is normal after a catheterization, but should continue to be monitored.
CN: Physiological integrity; CNS: Reduction of risk potential; CL: Application

3. 3. The elasticity of the lungs is lost for clients with emphysema, who can't tolerate lying flat because the abdominal organs compress the lungs. The best position is one with the head slightly elevated. The rate of oxygen delivery shouldn't be increased or decreased without an order from the physician. Increasing oxygen flow on a client with emphysema may also suppress the hypoxic drive to breathe. Positioning the client on his left side with the head of the bed flat would decrease oxygenation.
CN: Physiological integrity; CNS: Physiological adaptation; CL: Application

4. A 40-year-old client is scheduled to have elective facial surgery later in the morning. The nurse notes the pulse rate is 130 beats/minute. The nurse suspects which reason best explains the tachycardia?
   1. Age
   2. Anxiety
   3. Exercise
   4. Pain

5. A thin client is sitting up in bed talking on the phone and has a blood pressure of 90/50 mm Hg. Which nursing action is correct?
   1. Increase fluids.
   2. Call the physician.
   3. Consider this a normal variation.
   4. Suspect orthostatic hypotension.

6. Which sign should alert a nurse to a potential problem in a client who has received morphine I.V. for postoperative pain?
   1. Heart rate 124 beats/minute
   2. Respiratory rate 8 breaths/minute
   3. Sleeping, but easily aroused
   4. Blood pressure 90/62 mm Hg

7. The vital signs of a 56-year-old client are: temperature, 98.6° F (37° C) orally; pulse, 80 beats/minute; respirations, 30 breaths/minute; and blood pressure, 118/78 mm Hg. Which interpretation by the nurse is correct?
   1. Pulse is above normal range.
   2. Temperature is above normal range.
   3. Respirations are above normal range.
   4. Blood pressure is above normal range.

4. 2. Anxiety tends to increase heart rate, temperature, and respirations. The normal heart rate for a client this age is 60 to 100 beats/minute. Exercise will increase the heart rate but most likely won't occur preoperatively. The client shouldn't be in any pain preoperatively.
CN: Physiological integrity; CNS: Physiological adaptation; CL: Application

5. 3. A thin client can have a blood pressure as low as 88/46 mm Hg and remain asymptomatic. Calling the physician with this information is inappropriate, as is increasing fluids. Orthostatic hypotension is a decrease in blood pressure and increase in heart rate that occur with a sudden change in position from lying to sitting. It might indicate some dehydration, but this client had been sitting up without symptoms for a while.
CN: Health promotion and maintenance; CNS: None; CL: Application

6. 2. Since morphine depresses the respiratory center of the brain, the nurse should alert the physician of a respiratory rate less than 10 breaths/minute. While a heart rate of 124 beats/minute is considered tachycardia, the nurse should further assess the client before calling the physician. Morphine shouldn't be given to a client who is sedated and not easily aroused. Morphine can cause hypotension, but the nurse should further assess the client before calling the physician because this may be the client's usual blood pressure.
CN: Physiological integrity; CNS: Pharmacological and parenteral therapies; CL: Analysis

7. 3. Normal vital signs for an adult client are: temperature, 96.6° to 99° F (36° to 37° C); pulse, 60 to 100 beats/minute; respirations, 16 to 20 breaths/minute; and blood pressure, 90–120/60–80 mm Hg.
CN: Health promotion and maintenance; CNS: None; CL: Analysis

8. A client with type 1 diabetes mellitus is confused, weak, diaphoretic, and has palpitations. What action should the nurse take first?
1. Administer glucagon intramuscularly (I.M.) or subcutaneously (subQ).
2. Give an intravenous (I.V.) bolus of dextrose 50%.
3. Provide 15 to 20 g of a fast-acting oral carbohydrate.
4. Inject 10 units of fast-acting insulin subcutaneously.

9. Which nursing action is correct for performing tracheal suctioning?
1. Apply suction during insertion of the catheter.
2. Limit suctioning to 10 to 15 seconds' duration.
3. Resterilize the suction catheter in alcohol after use.
4. Repeat suctioning intervals every 15 minutes until clear.

10. While performing nasopharyngeal suction, a nurse notes a client's oxygen saturation reading is 86% by pulse oximeter. Which action should the nurse take?
1. Stop suctioning and give oxygen to the client.
2. Withdraw the suction catheter and tell the client to cough several times.
3. Continue suctioning for 10 to 15 more seconds and then withdraw the suction catheter.
4. Keep the suction catheter inserted and wait a few seconds before beginning suctioning.

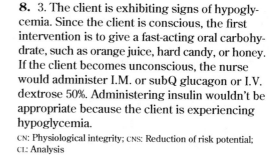

Ten done already! Good job!

11. Two hours after starting total enteral nutrition (TEN) through a nasogastric tube, a client starts to have abdominal distention. Which action should the nurse take first?
1. Aspirate stomach contents.
2. Reposition the tube.
3. Place client in supine position.
4. Stop the feeding.

8. 3. The client is exhibiting signs of hypoglycemia. Since the client is conscious, the first intervention is to give a fast-acting oral carbohydrate, such as orange juice, hard candy, or honey. If the client becomes unconscious, the nurse would administer I.M. or subQ glucagon or I.V. dextrose 50%. Administering insulin wouldn't be appropriate because the client is experiencing hypoglycemia.
CN: Physiological integrity; CNS: Reduction of risk potential; CL: Analysis

9. 2. The length of time a client should be able to tolerate the suction procedure is 10 to 15 seconds. Any longer may cause hypoxia. Suctioning during insertion can cause trauma to the mucosa and removes oxygen from the respiratory tract. Suctioning intervals with supplemental oxygen between suctions is performed after at least 1-minute intervals to allow the client to rest. Suction catheters are disposed of after each use and are cleansed in normal saline solution after each pass.
CN: Physiological integrity; CNS: Physiological adaptation; CL: Application

10. 1. The pulse oximeter reading indicates the client isn't oxygenating well, so the nurse must stop suctioning and give oxygen to increase the saturation. The normal range for oxygen saturation is 90% to 100%. Suctioning draws air as well as secretions from the lungs, reducing oxygen saturation in the blood. Withdrawing the suction catheter will stop the removal of oxygen, but coughing will delay an increase in saturation. Further suctioning will reduce the oxygen level even more. The suction catheter occupies space in the airway, making it harder for the client to breathe when it's left in place.
CN: Physiological integrity; CNS: Physiological adaptation; CL: Application

11. 4. Clients receiving TEN are at risk for abdominal distention due to rapid feeding or delayed emptying of the stomach contents. The first action would be to stop the feeding to prevent further distention and then continue to assess the distention's cause. Aspirating the stomach contents and repositioning the tube may be necessary, but are not the priority. A client receiving a nasogastric tube feeding should be placed in an upright or Fowler's position, not supine, to prevent the risk of aspiration.
CN: Physiological integrity; CNS: Basic care and comfort; CL: Application

12. Which step should a nurse take first when preparing to insert a nasogastric (NG) tube?
1. Wash hands.
2. Apply sterile gloves.
3. Apply a mask and gown.
4. Open all necessary kits and tubing.

13. As a nurse is inserting a nasogastric tube, the client begins to gag. Which action should the nurse take?
1. Remove the inserted tube and notify the physician of the client's status.
2. Stop the insertion, allow the client to rest, then continue inserting the tube.
3. Encourage the client to take deep breaths through the mouth while the tube is being inserted.
4. Pause until the gagging stops, tell the client to take a few sips of water and swallow as the tube is inserted.

14. Which step, if taken by a nurse after insertion of a nasogastric (NG) tube, could harm the client?
1. Affix the NG tube to the nose with tape.
2. Check tube placement by aspirating stomach contents using a piston syringe.
3. Check tube placement by instilling 100 ml of water into the tube to check for stomach filling.
4. Document in the chart the insertion, method used to check tube placement, and client's response to the procedure.

15. A new graduate nurse is assigned to a nursing unit. The nurse-manager notes that the graduate's skills are deficient. Which action is most appropriate for the nurse-manager to take?
1. Talk with the supervisor about terminating the new graduate.
2. Discuss with the graduate that a transfer to another unit is necessary.
3. Work with the graduate and develop a plan to improve the graduate's deficiencies.
4. Counsel the graduate that, if performance doesn't improve, the graduate will be terminated.

12. 1. The first intervention before a procedure is hand washing. Clean gloves are used because the mouth and nasopharynx aren't considered sterile. A mask and gown aren't required. Opening all the equipment is the next step before inserting the NG tube.
CN: Safe, effective care environment; CNS: Safety and infection control; CL: Application

13. 4. Swallowing helps advance the tube by causing the epiglottis to cover the opening of the trachea, thus helping to eliminate gagging and coughing. Removing the tube or stopping the insertion is unnecessary because gagging is an expected response to this procedure. Deep breathing opens the trachea, allowing the tube to possibly advance into the lungs.
CN: Safe, effective care environment; CNS: Safety and infection control; CL: Application

14. 3. Should the tube be located in the lungs, instilling water would flood the lungs, precipitating choking, coughing, hypoxemia and, possibly, pneumonia. Anchoring the tube after placement to the nose with tape or a manufactured device prevents the tube from becoming dislodged. Withdrawing stomach contents from the NG tube double-checks the correct placement. Documentation is required for any procedure.
CN: Safe, effective care environment; CNS: Management of care; CL: Application

15. 3. A principle of leadership involves mastery over ignorance by working with people. The leader needs to work with the new graduate and provide opportunities for the graduate to grow and develop. The other responses wouldn't give the new graduate the opportunity and support needed for improvement.
CN: Safe, effective care environment; CNS: Management of care; CL: Application

CN: Client needs category   CNS: Client needs subcategory   CL: Cognitive level

16. A client on a cardiac monitor has a heart rate of 170 beats/minute, with frequent premature contractions. Which nursing action is best?
1. Call the client's physician immediately.
2. See the client and make a full assessment.
3. Delegate one of the nurses' assistants to take the client's vital signs.
4. Notify the supervisor about the change in the client's condition.

16. 2. Because a change has occurred in the client's status, the nurse must assess the client first. This shouldn't be delegated to unlicensed personnel. Before the physician or supervisor is notified, a full assessment must be made.
CN: Safe, effective care environment; CNS: Management of care; CL: Application

17. A client is hospitalized with an acute sinus infection. Which assessment made by the nurse indicates serious complications?
1. Orbital edema
2. Nuchal rigidity
3. Fever of 102° F (39° C)
4. Frontal headache

17. 2. Nuchal rigidity indicates neurologic involvement, possibly meningitis. The other symptoms are typical of a sinus infection.
CN: Physiological integrity; CNS: Physiological adaptation; CL: Application

18. Which statement by a client who had nasal surgery indicates to the nurse that the client needs further teaching about postoperative care?
1. "I'll do frequent mouth care."
2. "I'll eat two oranges a day."
3. "I'll eat two bananas a day."
4. "I'll drink at least 8 glasses of fluid a day."

18. 3. After nasal surgery, the client shouldn't strain or bear down as this will increase the risk for bleeding. Bananas can cause severe constipation, which could lead to straining. The other interventions would be appropriate postoperative care for this client.
CN: Physiological integrity; CNS: Reduction of risk potential; CL: Analysis

19. The nurse is collecting a urine specimen from a client's indwelling urinary catheter. Which action should the nurse take?
1. Collect urine from the drainage collection bag.
2. Disconnect the catheter from the drainage tubing to collect urine.
3. Remove the indwelling catheter and insert a sterile straight catheter to collect urine.
4. Insert a sterile needle with syringe through a tubing drainage port cleaned with alcohol to collect the specimen.

19. 4. Wearing clean gloves, cleaning the port with alcohol, and then obtaining the specimen with a sterile needle ensures the specimen and the closed urinary drainage system won't be contaminated. A urine sample must be new urine, and the urine in the bag could be several hours old and growing bacteria. The urinary drainage system must be kept closed to prevent microorganisms from entering. A straight catheter is used to relieve urinary retention, obtain sterile urine specimens, measure the amount of postvoid residual urine, and empty the bladder for certain procedures. It isn't necessary to remove an indwelling catheter to obtain a sterile urine specimen unless the physician requests the whole system be changed.
CN: Safe, effective care environment; CNS: Safety and infection control; CL: Application

20. Which observation indicates to a nurse that a client understands his instructions on crutch walking?
   1. The client's axillae rest on the crutches.
   2. The client's hands bear the body weight.
   3. Crutches are 12″ (30.5 cm) in front of the feet.
   4. The client uses long strides when walking.

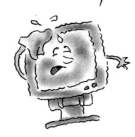

Don't sweat it! You're doing great!

20. 2. When using crutches, the client should bear weight on his hands. The axillae shouldn't rest on the crutches; there should be 2″ (5 cm) between the crutch and axilla. Crutches should be placed 6″ (15 cm) in front of the feet for stability. A short stride provides maximum safety and mobility.
CN: Physiological integrity; CNS: Basic care and comfort; CL: Application

21. A client recovering from a knee replacement has normal saline solution ordered to run at 125 ml/hour I.V. The I.V. bag was hung at 8:00 a.m. It's now 3:00 p.m., and 300 ml have been infused. A nurse has just come on her shift at 3:00 p.m. Which action is correct?
   1. Discontinue the I.V. infusion when the bag is complete.
   2. Instruct the client to increase his fluid intake.
   3. Speed up the rate of the I.V. fluids.
   4. Assess the intravenous site.

21. 4. At 125 ml/hour over 7 hours, 875 ml should have been infused. The I.V. fluid is 575 ml behind. The first action would be to make sure the site is not infiltrated before calling the physician for further fluid orders. The physician will determine how the I.V. fluids will be adjusted and will want to know why the client didn't get the prescribed fluids. The order is for I.V. fluids—not oral fluids—and the route change can only be authorized by a physician. Legally, the nurse can't change the rate of I.V. fluids.
CN: Safe, effective care environment; CNS: Management of care; CL: Application

22. A nurse is removing an indwelling urinary catheter from a client. Which action is appropriate?
   1. Wear sterile gloves.
   2. Cut the lumen of the balloon.
   3. Document the time of removal.
   4. Position the client on the left side.

22. 3. The client should void within 8 hours of the removal of an indwelling urinary catheter. Documenting the time of removal allows the nurse and physician to verify the duration of elapsed time since removal, thus contributing to continuity of care. Clean, disposable gloves are required because it isn't a sterile procedure. The catheter may retrograde into the bladder, requiring surgical removal, if the balloon is cut from the lumen and the catheter isn't secured. The client should be positioned comfortably on his back, and privacy should be provided.
CN: Safe, effective care environment; CNS: Safety and infection control; CL: Application

23. The nurse obtains a client's stool sample for occult blood. Which of the following diets can cause a false-positive test result?
   1. Red meat, horseradish, and turnips
   2. Dairy products, canned fruit, and pretzels
   3. Cheese, raw fruits, and vegetables
   4. Potatoes, orange juice, and decaffeinated coffee

23. 1. Consumption of red meat has caused false-positive readings. The client should also avoid poultry, fish, turnips, and horseradish. Avoid foods that are high in iron. The other foods don't cause false-positive readings.
CN: Physiological integrity; CNS: Basic care and comfort; CL: Application

CN: Client needs category   CNS: Client needs subcategory   CL: Cognitive level

24. A client complains of excessive flatulence. The nurse teaches the client about foods which, if consumed regularly, may be responsible for flatulence. Which selection of food, if made by the client, would indicate that the teaching has been effective?
1. Cauliflower
2. Ice cream
3. Steak
4. Potatoes

25. A nurse uses which technique when assisting a client with postoperative coughing and deep-breathing exercises?
1. Splint the incision and cough.
2. Splint the incision, take a deep breath, and then cough.
3. Lie prone, splint the incision, take a deep breath, and then cough.
4. Lie supine, splint the incision, take a deep breath, and then cough.

26. Which statement is an appropriate client goal, as written by the nurse?
1. The nurse will perform the client's bath by 3 p.m.
2. The client will bathe with assistance.
3. The nurse will perform the client's bath.
4. The client will bathe with assistance by discharge.

27. While helping a cooperative client with a diagnosis of acquired immunodeficiency syndrome with mouth care, the nurse should take which precaution?
1. Wear a mask, gown, and gloves.
2. Wear a gown and gloves.
3. Wear a mask with eye shield and gloves.
4. Wear gloves only.

24. 1. Foods that cause flatulence in some people may not produce flatulence in others. It all depends on the amount consumed, but cauliflower is the only food listed that usually results in flatulence.
CN: Physiological integrity; CNS: Basic care and comfort; CL: Application

25. 2. Splinting the incision with a pillow will protect the incision while the client coughs. Taking a deep breath will help open the alveoli, which promotes oxygen exchange and prevents atelectasis. Coughing and deep-breathing exercises are best accomplished in a sitting or semi-sitting position. Expectoration of secretions will be facilitated in a sitting position, as will splinting and taking deep breaths.
CN: Physiological integrity; CNS: Reduction of risk potential; CL: Application

26. 4. All goals should be client focused, allowing the client to understand what needs to be accomplished. Specify a time limit for when this task should be achieved. Be realistic, so the client may be successful in reaching the goal. The goal must be measurable so all staff can evaluate the client's progress. Nurse flexibility is an important attribute and necessary for reassessing needs and approaches for the client's optimal recovery. However, in the actual goal, specific criteria must be identified to allow all staff to work from the same data for achieving client goals.
CN: Safe, effective care environment; CNS: Management of care; CL: Application

27. 4. According to standard precautions, the nurse should wear gloves when coming in contact with a client's blood or body fluids. During mouth care with a cooperative client gloves are sufficient to protect the nurse. A mask is worn when airborne droplets of blood or body fluids are anticipated. A gown and mask with eye shield should be worn when splashing of body fluids are expected.
CN: Safe, effective care environment; CNS: Safety and infection control; CL: Application

28. The nurse would perform which action for developmentally-based care?
1. Provide books to a 9-year-old client.
2. Walk a 10-year-old client according to written orders.
3. Provide a pureed diet to a postoperative 13-year-old client.
4. Change a surgical dressing on a 15-year-old client every 4 hours as ordered.

29. A nurse has identified *Ineffective airway clearance* as a nursing diagnosis for a client with pneumonia. Which goal would be appropriate for this client?
1. The client will have clear breath sounds.
2. The client will have a respiratory rate of 32 breaths/minute.
3. The client will be pain-free.
4. The client will have a normal body temperature.

30. A client on complete bed rest complains of excessive flatulence. To best facilitate passage of flatus, the nurse places the client in which position?
1. Fowler's
2. Knee-chest
3. Semi-Fowler's
4. Trendelenburg's

31. The nurse is assisting with the delivery of a fetus where the mentum is the presenting part. Which graphic illustrates that fetal presentation?

1.

2.

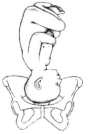

3.

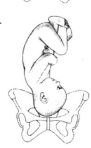

4.

You're at question 30 and looking good!

28. 1. Providing books to a 9-year-old client facilitates his reading skills and helps him grow developmentally. Changing a surgical dressing, walking a client, and providing a pureed diet are routine care tasks, which don't necessarily promote further development of the individual.
CN: Health promotion and maintenance; CNS: None; CL: Application

29. 1. Clear breath sounds in a client with pneumonia would indicate the airway is clear. Tachypnea would not indicate clear breath sounds and may occur when the client has difficulty clearing secretions. Being pain-free and having a normal body temperature are appropriate goals for a client with pneumonia but are not an indication that the airway is clear.
CN: Safe, effective care environment; CNS: Management of care; CL: Analysis

30. 2. Because gas rises, the knee-chest position facilitates the passage of flatus. Semi-Fowler's and Fowler's positions inhibit gas passage. In Trendelenburg's position, the client lies flat with his head lower than his feet.
CN: Physiological integrity; CNS: Basic care and comfort; CL: Application

31. 1. In the cephalic, or head-down, presentation, the fetus' position may be classified by the presenting skull landmark: mentum or chin (option 1), brow (option 2), sinciput (option 3), or vertex (option 4).
CN: Health promotion and maintenance; CNS: None; CL: Application

CN: Client needs category   CNS: Client needs subcategory   CL: Cognitive level

32. In which position should a nurse place a client with pneumonia when performing percussion and postural drainage to the left lower lobe?
1. Supine with the foot of the bed elevated
2. On the left side with the foot of the bed elevated
3. On the left side with the head of the bed elevated
4. Prone with the head of the bed elevated

33. The client is complaining of moderate pain. Which assessment by the nurse indicates a physiological response to pain?
1. Restlessness
2. Decreased pulse rate
3. Increased blood pressure
4. Protection of the painful area

34. A client with long-standing rheumatoid arthritis has frequent complaints of joint pain. The nurse's plan of treatment is based on the understanding that chronic pain is most effectively relieved when analgesics are administered in which way?
1. Conservatively
2. I.M.
3. On an as-needed basis
4. At regularly scheduled intervals

35. A nurse notes crackles in the lung bases and pedal edema during client assessment. Which factor is a common cause of fluid volume excess?
1. Prolonged fever
2. Hyperventilation
3. Excessive I.V. infusion
4. Fluid volume shifts secondary to vomiting

36. Which nursing intervention is correct for clients receiving I.V. therapy?
1. Change the tubing every 8 hours.
2. Monitor the flow rate at least every hour.
3. Change the I.V. catheter and entry site daily.
4. Increase the rate to catch up if the correct amount hasn't been infused at the end of the shift.

32. 1. To mobilize secretions from the left lower lobe the client should be positioned supine or on the right side. The foot of the bed should be elevated so that gravity can help mobilize secretions. Placing the client on the left side would put the left lobe in a low or dependent position. Elevating the head of the bed wouldn't use gravity to drain the lower lobes.
CN: Physiological integrity; CNS: Basic care and comfort; CL: Application

33. 3. Increased blood pressure is a physiological, or involuntary, response to moderate pain. Restlessness and protection of the painful area are behavioral responses. Decreased pulse rate occurs when pain is severe and deep.
CN: Physiological integrity; CNS: Physiological adaptation; CL: Analysis

34. 4. To control chronic pain and prevent cycled pain, regularly scheduled intervals are most effective. As-needed and conservative methods aren't effective means to manage chronic pain because the pain isn't relieved regularly. I.M. administration isn't practical on a long-term basis.
CN: Physiological integrity; CNS: Pharmacological and parenteral therapies; CL: Application

35. 3. Fluid volume excess can result from excess I.V. fluids, especially in a compromised client. Vomiting, fever, and hyperventilation will result in loss of body fluids, leading to a fluid volume deficit.
CN: Physiological integrity; CNS: Basic care and comfort; CL: Application

36. 2. Closely observing the rate of infusion prevents underhydration and overhydration. Tubing is changed according to facility policy but not at the frequency of every 8 hours. The I.V. catheter and entry site should be changed every 48 to 72 hours in most situations. Increasing the rate may lead to fluid overload.
CN: Physiological integrity; CNS: Pharmacological and parenteral therapies; CL: Application

37. A client is given instructions for a low-sodium diet. Which statement best shows the nurse that the client understands the diet instruction?
1. "Meat, fish, and chicken are high in sodium."
2. "I'll miss eating fruits."
3. "I'll enjoy eating at restaurants more often now."
4. "I'll avoid dairy products, potato chips, and carrots."

38. To prevent aspiration in a client with impaired swallowing, the nurse should:
1. provide a straw for drinking liquids.
2. remove dentures before eating.
3. position the client at a 90-degree angle.
4. place food on the paralyzed side of the mouth.

39. A client must choose a meal that follows his diet orders of a high-calorie, high-protein, low-sodium, and low-potassium diet. Which choice indicates to the nurse that the client understands the dietary guidelines?
1. Halibut, salad, rice, and instant coffee
2. Crab, beets, spinach, and baked potato
3. Salmon, rice, green beans, sourdough bread, coffee, and ice cream
4. Sirloin steak, salad, baked potato with butter, and chocolate ice cream

40. A client with terminal cancer tells the nurse, "I've given up. I have no hope left. I'm ready to die." Which response is most therapeutic?
1. "You've given up hope?"
2. "We should talk about dying to a social worker."
3. "You should talk to your physician about your fears of dying so soon."
4. "Now, you shouldn't give up hope. There are cures for cancer found every day."

37. 4. Dairy products, potato chips, carrots, and restaurant food are all high in sodium. Meat, fish, chicken, and fruits aren't.
CN: Physiological integrity; CNS: Basic care and comfort; CL: Application

38. 3. When feeding a client with impaired swallowing, the nurse should position the client at a 90-degree angle to reduce the risk of aspiration. Straws shouldn't be used because they increase the risk of aspiration by sending liquids directly to the back of the mouth. Dentures should be well-fitting and in place for eating. If one side of the mouth is paralyzed, food should be placed on the unaffected side.
CN: Physiological integrity; CNS: Basic care and comfort; CL: Application

39. 3. The best choice of these meals is salmon with rice and green beans, which is high in protein, and the sourdough bread and ice cream add calories. Halibut, instant coffee, and potatoes are high in potassium, and beets are high in sodium.
CN: Health promotion and maintenance; CNS: None; CL: Application

You're more than halfway finished! You're amazing!

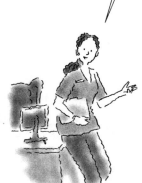

40. 1. The use of reflection invites the client to talk more about his concerns. Deferring the conversation to a social worker or physician closes the conversation. Telling the client the cure for cancer is right around the corner gives false hope.
CN: Psychosocial integrity; CNS: None; CL: Analysis

CN: Client needs category CNS: Client needs subcategory CL: Cognitive level

41. Which instruction should a nurse include in the teaching plan for a client with a platelet count of 25,000 mm³ and petechial rash on the legs, arms, and neck?
   1. Take an iron supplement daily.
   2. Take acetaminophen rather than aspirin for headache.
   3. Stay away from crowds during the flu season.
   4. Avoid fresh salads.

42. Which laboratory value for a newly diagnosed client with diabetes should the nurse report to the physician?
   1. pH, 7.45
   2. Sodium, 118 mEq/L
   3. Glucose, 120 mg/dl
   4. Potassium, 3.9 mEq/L

43. A client is 2 days postoperative from a femoral popliteal bypass. The nurse's assessment finds the client's left leg cold and pale. Which action has priority?
   1. Check distal pulses.
   2. Notify the physician.
   3. Elevate the foot of the bed.
   4. Wrap the leg in a warm blanket.

44. The nurse can administer which mediation through a nasogastric (NG) tube?
   1. Enteric coated aspirin
   2. Acetaminophen
   3. Regular insulin
   4. Sublingual nitroglycerine

41. 2. The client with thrombocytopenia has a low platelet count and should avoid products containing aspirin since they may increase the risk of bleeding. Iron supplements would be helpful in the client with anemia. Staying away from crowds and avoiding fresh salads to reduce the risk of infection would be important for the client with leukopenia.
CN: Physiological integrity; CNS: Reduction of risk potential; CL: Analysis

42. 2. The normal range for sodium is 135 to 145 mEq/L. The rest of the results are within normal limits.
CN: Physiological integrity; CNS: Reduction of risk potential; CL: Analysis

43. 1. The client has arterial disease and had vascular surgery. The nurse must assess the client for complications. A potential problem would be a clot at the surgical site, so the nurse must assess circulation by checking for distal pulses. Before the physician is notified, the nurse should determine if distal pulses are present. Elevating the foot of the bed would promote venous return but decrease arterial blood flow and shouldn't be done. The leg can be covered lightly after circulation is assessed.
CN: Physiological integrity; CNS: Physiological adaptation; CL: Application

44. 2. Most oral medications can be given through an NG tube because they're intended for passage into the stomach. Some oral drugs have special coatings intended to keep the pill intact until it passes into the small intestine; these enteric-coated pills shouldn't be crushed and put through an NG tube. Some parenteral medications, such as insulin, may be destroyed by gastric juices. Sublingual means under the tongue and parenteral means I.V., I.M., and subcutaneous.
CN: Physiological integrity; CNS: Pharmacological and parenteral therapies; CL: Application

45. The nurse knows if a client requires oxygen delivery at a FiO_2 of 92%, the appropriate system would be:
1. Face tent
2. Venturi mask
3. Nasal cannula
4. Mask with reservoir bag

45. 4. A mask with a reservoir bag administers 70% to 100% oxygen at flow rates of 8 to 10 L/minute. A face tent maximum delivery is 22% to 34%, the Venturi mask maximum rate is 24% to 55%, and the nasal cannula maximum rate is 44% at 6 L/minute.
CN: Physiological integrity; CNS: Pharmacological and parenteral therapies; CL: Analysis

46. The client has returned from the operating room with the nursing diagnosis of *Acute pain*. The nurse knows that the best means of providing comfort would be to administer:
1. morphine sulfate 10 mg intramuscularly (IM).
2. morphine sulfate 0.2 mg/ml via patient controlled analgesia (PCA).
3. Dilaudid 2 mg intravenously (IV) every 2 hours.
4. Percocet 5 mg orally (PO) every 4–6 hours.

46. 2. Clients who have ready access to an analgesic are more likely to medicate themselves before the pain becomes severe and thus may require reduced amounts of medication. Having control over drug administration also reduces anxiety, which helps to relieve pain.
CN: Physiological integrity; CNS: Pharmacological and parenteral therapies; CL: Application

47. A client with difficulty breathing has a respiratory rate of 34 breaths/minute and seems very anxious. He's refusing all his medications, claiming they're making him worse. Which nursing action is best?
1. Notify the physician of the status of this client.
2. Withhold the medication until the next scheduled dose.
3. Encourage the client to take some of his medications.
4. Put the medicine in applesauce to give it without the client's knowledge.

47. 1. Notifying the physician of the client's condition and his refusal to take his medications allows the physician to decide what alternatives should be instituted. Withholding a medication requires the physician to be notified. Even if the client takes some of the medications, the physician will still need to be notified. It needs to be explored why the client believes the medications are making him worse. Giving medications in applesauce destroys trust between the nurse and client.
CN: Physiological integrity; CNS: Pharmacological and parenteral therapies; CL: Application

48. Which statement is an example of a key element in the nursing care plan?
1. Advance diet to regular as tolerated.
2. Ambulate 30′ (9 m) with walker by discharge.
3. Give furosemide (Lasix) 40 mg I.V. now.
4. Discontinue I.V. fluids when tolerating oral fluids.

48. 2. Ambulating 30′ with a walker by discharge is a measurable expected outcome or goal, a key element of a nursing care plan. Other key elements include nursing diagnoses and interventions. The other options are physician's orders, not key elements of care plans.
CN: Safe, effective care environment; CNS: Management of care; CL: Application

CN: Client needs category   CNS: Client needs subcategory   CL: Cognitive level

49. A client who was recently hospitalized has a nursing diagnosis of *Constipation related to medical regime*. Which medication may contribute to this problem?
 1. Folic acid
 2. Iron
 3. Potassium
 4. Vitamin E

30, 40, 50 down... and only 25 more to go!

49. 2. Iron may cause constipation when supplements are taken at 100% of the RDA. Folic acid, potassium, and vitamin E don't increase the likelihood of constipation.
CN: Physiological integrity; CNS: Pharmacological and parenteral therapies; CL: Application

50. A client had an appendectomy 24 hours ago. Which nursing goal is appropriate for this client?
 1. The client will be able to walk in the hallway.
 2. The client will be able to attend physical therapy.
 3. The client will be able to accomplish all activities of daily living.
 4. The client will be able to state the rationale for all postoperative medications.

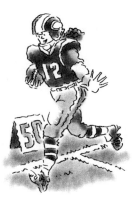

50. 1. A 24-hour postoperative client is expected to be able to walk in the hallway. A client who just had an appendectomy shouldn't need physical therapy unless deconditioning was evident. At 24 hours, a client should begin to assume responsibility for activities of daily living, but shouldn't necessarily be responsible for all activities. It's too early to expect a client to state the rationale for all postoperative medications, especially if the client is elderly.
CN: Physiological integrity; CNS: Basic care and comfort; CL: Application

51. Which nursing discharge instruction has the highest priority for a client going home with a full leg cast?
 1. Activity restrictions
 2. Proper nutrition
 3. Weight-bearing limitations
 4. Reporting signs of impaired circulation

51. 4. The nurse should include all these instructions in the teaching plan; however, the highest priority is teaching the signs of impaired circulation to prevent permanent neurovascular damage, including loss of the leg.
CN: Physiological integrity; CNS: Reduction of risk potential; CL: Analysis

52. During an initial nursing assessment, a nurse uses open-ended questions to gather data. Which statement would the nurse make, or which question would the nurse ask?
 1. "Tell me how things have been going for you."
 2. "Have you been feeling good?"
 3. "Tell me what you mean when you say you've been feeling funny."
 4. "I'd like to ask you more about your chest pain."

52. 1. "Tell me how things have been going for you" is an open-ended question that encourages the client to speak and express concerns. Asking the client if he feels good is a closed-ended question that only requires a "yes" or "no" response. The third option is seeking clarification of a statement made by the client. The fourth option is a focused question designed to help the nurse collect information on a specific health concern.
CN: Psychosocial integrity; CNS: None; CL: Application

53. A registered nurse (RN) is supervising an unlicensed care provider. Which principle would the nurse follow when delegating tasks?
1. The RN must directly supervise all delegated tasks.
2. After a task is delegated, it's no longer the RN's responsibility.
3. The RN is responsible for delegating tasks to adjunct personnel.
4. Follow-up with a delegated task is necessary only if the assistive personnel are untrustworthy.

54. An elderly client had recent surgery and is on bed rest. When planning care for the client, which nursing intervention is included in the care plan?
1. Daily assessment of the wound site
2. Foot and ankle range-of-motion (ROM) exercises
3. Wound cleaning with hydrogen peroxide
4. Coughing and deep breathing in the prone position

55. A client receiving phenothiazine has become restless and fidgety and has been pacing the hallway continuously for the past hour. This behavior suggests to the nurse that the client may be experiencing which adverse reaction to phenothiazine?
1. Dystonia
2. Akathisia
3. Parkinsonian effects
4. Tardive dyskinesia

56. A client who had his gallbladder removed 2 days ago now complains of pain in the right calf. Which nursing response has priority?
1. Assess the leg for swelling and redness.
2. Instruct the client to flex his knee and hip.
3. Apply a warm compress and call the physician.
4. Gently massage the calf and notify the physician.

53. 3. The RN must delegate tasks that are within the scope of practice of the unlicensed personnel. The RN need not directly supervise all delegated tasks as that would negate the benefits of delegation. Even when the task is delegated, the RN retains responsibility for the successful completion of the task. The RN must always follow up with the assistive personnel to ensure the task was completed appropriately, not only in instances of mistrust.

CN: Safe, effective care environment; CNS: Management of care; CL: Application

54. 2. Foot and ankle ROM exercises are standard protocol for clients who remain in bed for an extended period of time. ROM exercises promote blood flow to the area, prevent atrophy, and lessen the potential for edema. The wound site should be assessed every shift. Wound cleaning with hydrogen peroxide isn't generally recommended. Coughing and deep breathing aren't generally recommended in the prone position.

CN: Physiological integrity; CNS: Reduction of risk potential; CL: Application

55. 2. The client's behavior suggests akathisia—an adverse effect of phenothiazines. Dystonia appears as excessive salivation, difficulty speaking, and involuntary movements of the face, neck, arms and legs. Parkinsonian effects include a shuffling gait, hand tremors, drooling, rigidity, and loose arm movements. Tardive dyskinesia is characterized by odd facial and tongue movements.

CN: Physiological integrity; CNS: Reduction of risk potential; CL: Application

56. 1. Pain in the calf is a symptom of possible deep vein thrombosis. The nurse must assess further. Assessing the client for redness and swelling would be the next intervention. Making the client flex his knee and hip won't help assess for the presence of a clot. Warm compresses may be ordered after a diagnosis of deep vein thrombosis is made. Never massage the calf muscle because the clot could be dislodged.

CN: Physiological integrity; CNS: Reduction of risk potential; CL: Analysis

CN: Client needs category   CNS: Client needs subcategory   CL: Cognitive level

57. Which goal will the nurse make the highest priority in a client with a new tracheostomy?
  1. Developing an effective means of communication
  2. Maintaining a patent airway
  3. Preventing infection
  4. Gaining independence in self-care

58. Which statement by a client with chronic arterial disease indicates to the nurse further teaching is needed?
  1. "I'm going to stop smoking."
  2. "I'm going to have the podiatrist check my feet."
  3. "I'm going to keep the heat in my house at 80° F."
  4. "I'm going to walk short distances every morning."

59. A registered nurse is in charge of eight clients. The nurse has a licensed practical nurse (LPN) and a client care assistant working under her. Which activity should the nurse assign to herself rather than delegate to the staff?
  1. Consoling a grieving visitor
  2. Assessing a newly admitted client
  3. Irrigating a Salem sump to continuous drainage
  4. Giving a tap water enema to a preoperative client

60. A 6-year-old client needs diabetic teaching. Which factor is considered when the nurse plans the teaching?
  1. Another child with diabetes can teach the client.
  2. The child can teach his parents after the nurse teaches him.
  3. The child and parents should be recipients of teaching.
  4. Teaching should be directed to the parents, who then can teach the child.

57. 2. Maintaining a patent airway has the highest priority in a client with a new tracheostomy since drainage and edema can obstruct the airway. The other goals are also important but only after airway patency has been assured.
CN: Physiological integrity; CNS: Reduction of risk potential; CL: Analysis

58. 3. Clients with peripheral vascular disease need to be at a comfortable temperature because of impaired circulation. Having the heat at 80° F is too warm. The other choices are all appropriate interventions for a client with peripheral vascular disease.
CN: Physiological integrity; CNS: Reduction of risk potential; CL: Application

59. 2. Assessment of a new admission can't be delegated to an LPN. Consoling a visitor and giving a tap water enema are within the scope of practice of an LPN and client care assistant. Irrigation of a Salem sump is under the scope of practice of an LPN.
CN: Safe, effective care environment; CNS: Management of care; CL: Application

You're almost there! Keep going!

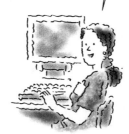

60. 3. The parents and child should participate in the nurse's teaching to ensure accuracy of teaching and that the child has educated adult caregivers. The school-aged child shouldn't be the sole provider of teaching to the parents. Another school-aged child couldn't be entrusted to teach this child, although their input would be valuable. Parents should be included in the teaching plan but shouldn't be responsible for the teaching.
CN: Health promotion and maintenance; CNS: None; CL: Application

61. Parents of a toddler are having problems putting him to bed at night. Which recommendation by a nurse is most appropriate?
   1. Stop the afternoon naps.
   2. Allow the toddler to have a tantrum for ½ hour.
   3. Encourage the parents to develop nighttime rituals.
   4. Allow the toddler to have some control over bedtime.

62. After abdominal surgery for repair of an aortic aneurysm, a client may show maladaptive coping behavior in response to body changes related to the surgery. Which nursing intervention is best?
   1. Let the client express his feelings.
   2. Explain that a psychological referral would be beneficial.
   3. Instruct the client on how to use positive coping strategies.
   4. Encourage the client to participate in diversionary activities.

63. A new nurse graduate has started at the medical center and is assigned to a preceptor. The preceptor and other staff report that the nurse is uncooperative and unwilling to take direction. Which action by the preceptor is appropriate?
   1. Explain the behavior won't be tolerated.
   2. Ask the nurse why she wants to work here.
   3. Reestablish goals with the nurse.
   4. Begin the disciplinary process with this nurse.

64. A client with a history of bipolar disorder rushes into the mental health clinic waiting room scantily dressed and makes loud, obscene remarks to other clients. Which response by the nurse has priority?
   1. Encourage the other clients to ignore the behavior.
   2. Confront the behavior and make the client take a seat.
   3. Tell the client to sit down and stop upsetting the others.
   4. Quietly escort the client to a private area and help put on a gown.

61. 3. Rituals are extremely important for toddlers to feel secure and relaxed. Allowing a toddler to make small decisions, such as choosing the order of the ritual and color of pajamas, will give him the feeling of some control. Stopping the naps may be helpful, depending on the toddler's needs. The toddler must clearly understand that tantrums won't get him what he wants.
CN: Health promotion and maintenance; CNS: None; CL: Application

62. 1. Allowing verbalization of feelings is the most therapeutic nursing intervention. Making a referral may help, but initially the client should be allowed to express his feelings. Giving advice may stop therapeutic communication. Providing diversionary activities doesn't foster effective coping.
CN: Psychosocial integrity; CNS: None; CL: Analysis

63. 3. This is a new graduate in orientation and the preceptor should help this nurse learn the responsibilities and routines and reestablish goals. If the behavior continues, the nurse may need career counseling. This person isn't experienced and therefore shouldn't be reprimanded. Asking the nurse "why" in relation to working is inappropriate; it's the behavior that's creating the problem. This nurse shouldn't be disciplined as an initial step.
CN: Safe, effective care environment; CNS: Management of care; CL: Application

64. 4. The client with bipolar disorder is highly excitable. The nurse needs to be firm yet distracting, and this is best done in a private area, which also preserves the client's dignity. Having the others ignore the client won't alter the problem. Confronting the behavior isn't desired as this client lacks judgment and insight. Telling the client to sit down may cause the client to be more resistive and even heighten the behavior.
CN: Psychosocial integrity; CNS: None; CL: Analysis

CN: Client needs category   CNS: Client needs subcategory   CL: Cognitive level

65. A nurse is reviewing treatment of hypercyanotic spells (tet spells) with the parents of a 4-month-old client being discharged from the hospital. Which discharge instruction is correct?
1. "Calm the baby down by holding her and placing her knees up to her chest."
2. "Call 911 immediately and begin cardiopulmonary resuscitation (CPR) on the baby."
3. "You'll need to administer four back blows to the baby if she begins having a tet spell."
4. "You don't need to worry about these spells yet because the baby is too young. You'll need to watch for them when she becomes more mobile."

66. Which nursing intervention should a nurse use when caring for a client with gout?
1. Administer antibiotic.
2. Restrict fluid intake.
3. Encourage a low-purine diet.
4. Administer opioids.

67. The nurse is evaluating a client who is 2 days post crush injury to his right leg. Which symptom is a late indicator of compartment syndrome?
1. Sudden decrease in pain
2. Swelling in toes or fingers
3. Inability to move fingers or toes
4. Diminished distal pulses

68. A client with an arm cast complains of severe pain in the affected extremity and decreased sensation and motion are noted. Swelling in the fingers is also increased. Which nursing intervention has priority?
1. Elevate the arm.
2. Remove the cast.
3. Give an analgesic.
4. Call the physician.

65. 1. Tet spells are acute episodes of cyanosis and hypoxia that occur when the infant's oxygen demand exceeds the available supply. They may occur when the infant is crying or eating. Tet spells are emergency situations that require immediate intervention. Begin by calming the infant down and placing the infant in the knee-chest position, which increases systemic vascular resistance by limiting venous return. This decreases the right to left shunting and improves oxygenation. CPR won't calm the infant down or improve oxygenation. Back blows are given to infants who have something lodged in their trachea.
CN: Physiological integrity; CNS: Reduction of risk potential; CL: Application

66. 3. A low-purine diet decreases uric acid formation and should be encouraged. Antibiotics aren't used to treat gout. Fluid intake should be encouraged to flush out the uric acid. Anti-inflammatory medications are used during acute phases, but because this is a long-term condition, opioids aren't generally given.
CN: Physiological integrity; CNS: Reduction of risk potential; CL: Application

67. 4. Compartment syndrome is a complication of a cast that places pressure on the blood vessels and nerves to the extremity. Symptoms include pain not relieved by analgesics and swelling of the extremity. A late symptom is a change in skin color with diminished distal pulses. After a fracture, some swelling and pain result, but pulses need to be monitored, as well as color, sensation, and movement.
CN: Physiological integrity; CNS: Reduction of risk potential; CL: Analysis

68. 4. The cast may be too tight and may need to be split or removed by the physician. The arm should already be elevated. Notify the physician when circulation, sensation, or motion is impaired. Giving analgesics wouldn't be the first step as they may mask the signs of a serious problem.
CN: Physiological integrity; CNS: Reduction of risk potential; CL: Application

69. The nurse is performing preoperative teaching on a 4-year-old scheduled for cardiac catheterization. Which characteristic is correct for preoperative teaching?

1. Basic and performed close to the implementation of the procedure
2. Done several days before the procedure so the child will have time to prepare
3. Detailed in regard to the actual procedure so the child will know exactly what to expect
4. Directed at the child's parents because the child is too young to understand the procedure

70. A registered nurse is directing unlicensed personnel to draw the morning blood work for a 4-year-old child in the hospital. The nurse emphasizes the procedure is to be done in the treatment room. Which rationale is correct?

1. The procedure will be faster.
2. The child won't fear painful procedures done while he's in his bed.
3. The child can only be restrained on the examination table.
4. The parents won't observe the procedure and upset the child.

71. A client tells a nurse, "My medical illness is the result of something bad I did to someone in the past." Which response by the nurse is the most appropriate?

1. "What did you do wrong?"
2. "Let's talk about your concerns."
3. "That's silly! Don't believe that!"
4. "You're suffering from a psychiatric delusion. Relax, it will end soon."

72. A client on a psychiatric unit asks a nurse about the medications another client takes. Which response is best?

1. "How close are the two of you?"
2. "I can't give you that information, I must protect her privacy."
3. "Let me ask her if it's OK for me to tell you about her condition and medications."
4. "The client is taking insulin for her diabetes and digoxin for her heart condition."

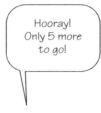

Hooray!
Only 5 more
to go!

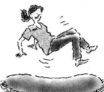

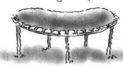

69. 1. Four-year-old children are in Piaget's cognitive stage of preoperational thought. Their thinking is concrete and tangible, and they're unable to make deductions or generalizations and are egocentric. They don't have a concept for the future so explanations need to be done close to the time of the procedure, not days in advance. They need simple explanations of procedures in relationship to how the procedure will affect them. A 4-year-old child is old enough to understand basic teaching close to the implementation of the procedure.
CN: Health promotion and maintenance; CNS: None; CL: Application

70. 2. This implementation is based on the concept of "atraumatic care" and growth and development principles. Small children need to have a safe zone in their beds to relax and rest in their rooms. The treatment room is used instead. It won't be faster to draw blood in the treatment room; it would take the same amount of time regardless of where it's done. The child could be restrained in his room, but it isn't appropriate. Parental support is important and needs to be encouraged during stressful and painful procedures.
CN: Psychosocial integrity; CNS: None; CL: Application

71. 2. Asking the client to talk about his concerns allows an opportunity for the nurse to clarify issues. Calling the client silly or asking the client what he did wrong would likely escalate the client's concerns. Telling the client it will end soon gives false reassurance.
CN: Psychosocial integrity; CNS: None; CL: Application

72. 2. Revealing one client's medication to another client is violating procedures of client confidentiality. Asking the client the nature of his relationship to the other client won't help the client understand the purpose of protecting confidentiality. Seeking the client's permission to release confidential information is an inappropriate action. Assuring the client that the hospital has an obligation to protect not only his confidentiality but that of others will provide the client with a sense of comfort.
CN: Safe, effective care environment; CNS: Management of care; CL: Application

CN: Client needs category   CNS: Client needs subcategory   CL: Cognitive level

73. A client's goal is to interact verbally at least once in each group therapy session by a certain date. The client attended the group session, maintained eye contact with the group members, followed the conversation nonverbally as indicated by head nodding, and spoke once to the group leader by giving a one-word answer. Which judgment by a nurse about goal attainment is correct?
1. The goal was partially met.
2. The goal was completely met.
3. The goal was completely unmet.
4. New problems or nursing diagnoses have developed.

73. 1. This goal was partially met because the client must verbally participate more in the group. For a goal to be completely met, the client must show the subjective and objective data indicating the goal has been clearly attained. A completely unmet goal indicates the client's complete lack of behavior change and absence of subjective and objective data to indicate the achievement of the goal. In this case, no new problems or new nursing diagnoses were evident.
CN: Psychosocial integrity; CNS: None; CL: Analysis

74. A client is prescribed heparin 6,000 units subcutaneously every 12 hours for deep vein thrombosis prophylaxis. The pharmacy dispenses a vial containing 10,000 units/ml. How many milliliters of heparin should a nurse administer? Record your answer using one decimal place.

_____ milliliters

74. 0.6. The following formula is used to calculate drug dosages: Dose on hand/Quantity on hand = Dose desired/X. The dose dispensed by the pharmacy is 10,000 units/1 ml and the desired dose is 6,000 units. The nurse should use the following equations: 10,000 units/1 ml = 6,000 units/X; 10,000 units (X) = 6,000 units (ml)/10,000 units; X = 0.6 ml.
CN: Physiological integrity; CNS: Pharmacological and parenteral therapies; CL: Analysis

75. A client is prescribed lisinopril (Zestril) for treatment of hypertension. He asks the nurse about possible adverse effects. The nurse should teach him about which common adverse effects of angiotensin converting enzyme (ACE) inhibitors? Select all that apply:
1. Constipation
2. Dizziness
3. Headache
4. Hyperglycemia
5. Hypotension
6. Impotence

75. 2, 3, 5. Dizziness, headache, and hypotension are all common adverse effects of lisinopril and other ACE inhibitors. Lisinopril may cause diarrhea, not constipation. It isn't known to cause hyperglycemia or impotence.
CN: Physiological integrity; CNS: Pharmacological and parenteral therapies; CL: Application

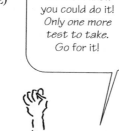

You're terrific! I knew you could do it! Only one more test to take. Go for it!

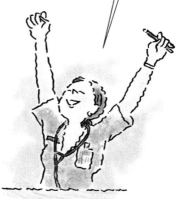

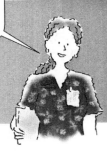

This is the LAST comprehensive test. Good luck! I know you're ready for it.

COMPREHENSIVE
Test 6

1. The nurse is teaching clients about hypertension and the importance of risk factors. Which client response identifying a nonmodifiable risk factor indicates that the teaching has been effective?
1. High sodium intake
2. Sedentary lifestyle
3. Tobacco use
4. Family history

2. A client experienced an acute inferior myocardial infarction at a community hospital. After antithrombolytic therapy fails, the physician wants to transfer the client to another hospital for emergency cardiac catheterization. Which member of the health care team must accompany the client?
1. Physician
2. Paramedic
3. Registered nurse (RN)
4. Licensed practical nurse (LPN)

3. A 56-year-old client with heart failure is allergic to sulfa-based medications. Which type of diuretic should be used cautiously?
1. Osmotic diuretics
2. Thiazide and thiazide-like diuretics
3. Potassium-sparing diuretics
4. Carbonic anhydrase inhibitors

4. A client with heart failure says he sleeps with two pillows because he experiences difficulty breathing when lying flat. The nurse documents which type of breathing?
1. Bradypnea
2. Dyspnea on exertion
3. Paroxysmal nocturnal dyspnea
4. Orthopnea

1. 4. Family history is a risk factor for hypertension that can't be modified. Risk factors that can be modified include high-sodium intake, sedentary lifestyle, and tobacco use.
CN: Health promotion and maintenance; CNS: None; CL: Application

2. 3. During transfer, the client must receive the same level of care that he received in the hospital; therefore, an RN must accompany him. It isn't necessary for a physician to accompany the client. A paramedic, although not required, will most likely accompany the nurse. An LPN is below the standard of care for this situation.
CN: Safe, effective care environment; CNS: Management of care; CL: Application

3. 2. Thiazide and thiazide-like diuretics are sulfonamide derivatives, so their use should be used cautiously in clients allergic to sulfa-based medications. Osmotic, potassium-sparing, and carbonic anhydrase inhibitor diuretics can be safely administered to these clients.
CN: Physiological integrity; CNS: Pharmacological and parenteral therapies; CL: Application

4. 4. A client with orthopnea has shortness of breath when lying flat, so he prefers sleeping with the upper body elevated. Bradypnea is decreased but regular breathing. Dyspnea on exertion occurs when the client has difficulty breathing with activity. Paroxysmal nocturnal dyspnea occurs when the client awakens at night and feels short of breath.
CN: Health promotion and maintenance; CNS: None; CL: Application

CN: Client needs category   CNS: Client needs subcategory   CL: Cognitive level

5. During an initial assessment of a neonate, the nurse notes a respiratory rate of 62 breaths/minute. How should the nurse intervene?
   1. Notify the physician immediately.
   2. Do nothing; this is a normal respiratory rate for a neonate.
   3. Position the isolette so the neonate's head is elevated.
   4. Prepare for emergency endotracheal (ET) intubation.

6. During a neonate's 1-month checkup, the pediatrician flexes the neonate's legs to right angles at the hips and knees, and abducts both hips until the knees touch the table. Which statement describes the purpose of this test?
   1. To check the neonate's flexibility
   2. To assess leg strength
   3. To check for developmental dysplasia of the hip
   4. To examine the neonate for a hydrocele

7. At which age should a nurse initially screen for idiopathic juvenile scoliosis?
   1. 7 years
   2. 10 years
   3. 13 years
   4. 16 years

8. Which position is correct for scoliosis screening of a 10-year-old client?
   1. Facing away from the examiner, standing upright with his arms held out straight in front of his body
   2. Facing away from the examiner, bending forward in 50% flexion with his arms and head dangling
   3. Facing the examiner, standing upright with his arms held straight at his sides
   4. Sitting in a chair with feet flat on the floor and his back at a 90-degree angle

5. 2. A normal respiratory rate for a neonate is 30 to 80 breaths/minute, so notifying the physician or elevating the neonate's head isn't necessary. The nurse should prepare for ET intubation if the neonate has signs of imminent respiratory distress such as an expiratory grunt.
CN: Health promotion and maintenance; CNS: None; CL: Analysis

6. 3. This test assesses for developmental dysplasia of the hip. If dysplasia is present, the physician can see, feel, and sometimes hear a click. Although a neonate's flexibility and leg strength may be assessed at age 1 month, the examination techniques differ from those described here. To identify a hydrocele, the physician palpates the neonate's testes.
CN: Physiological integrity; CNS: Physiological adaptation; CL: Analysis

7. 2. Children should have initial screening at age 10—immediately before the adolescent growth spurt—when promontory signs of scoliosis may become apparent. By age 13, a child may have significantly developed scoliosis that requires surgery.
CN: Health promotion and maintenance; CNS: None; CL: Application

8. 2. Assessing a client's back for asymmetry, or a "razorback" hump, is best done with the client bending at the waist in 50% flexion with the arms and head dangling. This assessment can also be done with the arms hanging dependently at the sides so the examiner can check for asymmetry at the shoulders, waist folds, and space between the arms and waist.
CN: Health promotion and maintenance; CNS: None; CL: Application

9. Parents bring their infant to the clinic for a checkup after he was hospitalized with a new onset of type 1 diabetes mellitus. Which statement to the nurse indicates an understanding of their child's current situation?

   1. "The physician was wrong about the diagnosis because all of my child's fingersticks have been normal."
   2. "My child has experienced a honeymoon period, which could last 1 month to 1 year, and hasn't required any insulin injections."
   3. "Nobody in our family has diabetes, so how can my child have it?"
   4. "If our child lives a careful, sedentary lifestyle, she won't need as much insulin."

10. The nurse is preparing to administer an injection subcutaneously. Which graphic indicates the appropriate needle selection for this type of injection?

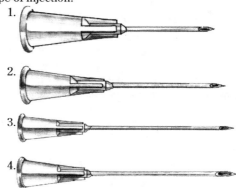

   1.
   2.
   3.
   4.

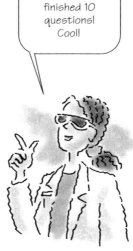

You've finished 10 questions! Cool!

9. 2. A honeymoon phase—in which injected insulin seems to wake up the islet cells and cause them to secrete insulin—is common with type 1 diabetes mellitus. This phase has given many parents false hope that their child has been cured. Type 1 diabetes isn't a genetic trait, and a sedentary lifestyle will increase the secondary effects of diabetes.

CN: Physiological integrity; CNS: Physiological adaptation; CL: Analysis

10. 2. When choosing a needle, consider its purpose as well as its gauge, bevel, and length. Graphic 2 indicates a subcutaneous needle which has a length of ½″ to ⅝″ long and medium bevel. The first graphic is of an intradermal needle, which has a length of ⅜″ to ⅝″ and short bevel. The third graphic is an intramuscular needle, which is 1″ to 3″ in length and medium bevel. The fourth graphic is an intravenous needle, which is 1″ to 3″ long with a long bevel.

CN: Physiological integrity; CNS: Pharmacological and parenteral therapies; CL: Application

11. Which intervention should a nurse include in the care plan for a 2-year-old child with Wilms' tumor?
  1. Tell the parents that surgery will be within 24 to 48 hours.
  2. Palpate the abdomen to monitor tumor size.
  3. Massage the abdomen to relieve pain.
  4. Place a tight binder around the abdomen for support.

12. Two days after undergoing a left thoracotomy, a client's temperature reaches 102° F (38.9° C). The nurse notifies the physician who orders two sets of blood cultures. Which amount of blood would the nurse obtain for cultures?
  1. 2 ml
  2. 5 ml
  3. 10 ml
  4. 20 ml

13. A charge nurse is developing the client-care assignments for the shift. Which client is most appropriately assigned to a licensed practical nurse (LPN)?
  1. A newly admitted client with stroke and do-not-resuscitate (DNR) status
  2. A client who underwent cerebral arteriography 1 hour ago
  3. A client who underwent carotid endarterectomy 4 hours ago
  4. A client who underwent craniotomy 3 days ago and has just been transferred from the intensive care unit (ICU)

14. A physician prescribes carbamazepine (Tegretol) 1,200 mg P.O. b.i.d. for a client with trigeminal neuralgia. Which action should the nurse take first?
  1. Administer the medication with meals.
  2. Encourage the client to promptly report unusual bleeding, bruising, fever, or chills.
  3. Question the order because the dose exceeds the recommended daily dose.
  4. Store the drug in a cool, dry place.

11. 1. The nurse tells the parents that the child will be scheduled for a nephrectomy within 24 to 48 hours because these tumors metastasize quickly. To reduce the risk of dissemination of cancer cells, the abdomen shouldn't be palpated or massaged. A tight binder may put pressure on the tumor, increasing the risk of dissemination and should, therefore, be avoided.
CN: Safe, effective care environment; CNS: Management of care; CL: Application

12. 3. When an adult client requires blood cultures, the nurse should draw 10 ml of blood; 5 ml should be injected into an anaerobic (without oxygen) bottle and 5 ml injected into an aerobic (with oxygen) bottle.
CN: Physiological integrity; CNS: Reduction of risk potential; CL: Application

13. 1. The most appropriate client to assign to the LPN is the newly admitted client with DNR status; typically, a newly admitted client is assigned to a registered nurse (RN) because the client requires frequent assessments. The client who recently underwent cerebral arteriography and the client who recently underwent carotid endarterectomy require frequent assessments by an RN. The client just transferred from the ICU has the potential for becoming unstable; therefore, an RN should care for this client.
CN: Safe, effective care environment; CNS: Management of care; CL: Analysis

14. 3. The first intervention by the nurse should be to question the order because it exceeds the recommended daily dose. Clients with trigeminal neuralgia should receive no more than 1,200 mg/day. After the nurse obtains an appropriate order, she should encourage the client to take the drug at equally spaced intervals with food to avoid GI distress. The nurse should also encourage the client to promptly report unusual bleeding, bruising, jaundice, dark urine, pale stools, abdominal pain, impotence, fever, chills, sore throat, mouth ulcers, edema, or disturbances in mood, alertness, or coordination. The drug should be stored in a cool, dry place.
CN: Physiological integrity; CNS: Pharmacological and parenteral therapies; CL: Analysis

15. Emergency medical system personnel have used the Cincinnati prehospital stroke scale to assess a client and have alerted the hospital that they're transporting a client with a possible stroke. The nurse plans to administer fibrinolytics within which time period?
1. 4 hours of the onset of symptoms
2. 60 minutes of arrival in the emergency department (ED)
3. 2 hours of arrival in the ED
4. 25 minutes of arrival in the ED

15. 2. The goal for initiating fibrinolytic therapy is within 60 minutes of arrival in the ED. Fibrinolytics must be administered within 3 hours of the onset of symptoms.
CN: Physiological integrity; CNS: Pharmacological and parenteral therapies; CL: Application

16. A client with an above-the-knee amputation visits the orthopedic surgeon for a follow-up. Which comment to the nurse would indicate the client is properly caring for the stump and prosthetic leg?
1. "I inspect the stump weekly to look for signs of redness, blistering, or abrasions."
2. "I put my prosthesis on before I get out of bed."
3. "I wash the stump every day with an antiseptic soap."
4. "I wipe out the socket of my prosthesis with a damp, soapy cloth weekly."

16. 2. The prosthesis should be applied upon rising in the morning. The stump and prosthesis should be inspected daily and cleaned daily with a mild soap. The prosthesis should be kept clean to prevent irritation or pressure areas from dirt or bacteria.
CN: Health promotion and maintenance; CNS: None; CL: Analysis

17. A nurse is caring for a client after a total knee replacement. The extremity was placed in a continuous passive motion (CPM) machine. Which action is one of the nurse's responsibilities?
1. Check the cycle and range-of-motion settings every morning.
2. Increase the degrees of flexion daily guided by client level of tolerance.
3. Decrease the degree of extension daily.
4. Turn the machine off when the client is eating a meal.

17. 4. The CPM machine can be turned off during meals to improve client comfort. The cycle and degrees of flexion should be checked every shift, and either the physician or physical therapist determines how and when the degrees of flexion can be increased. Usually, extension – as well as flexion – is increased, not decreased, on a regular basis.
CN: Physiological integrity; CNS: Basic care and comfort; CL: Application

CN: Client needs category   CNS: Client needs subcategory   CL: Cognitive level

18. A client has multiple myeloma. Which action should alert the nurse that he may be having difficulty coping with his prognosis?

1. He becomes tearful when discussing his condition.
2. He asks questions about his prognosis.
3. He shows concerns about his family.
4. He avoids any conversation concerning his health.

19. Which client is most likely to develop ankylosing spondylitis?

1. White female, age 16, with knee pain
2. Black male, age 50, with hip pain
3. Asian female, age 70, with chest pain
4. White male, age 23, with back pain

20. A client with pernicious anemia undergoes gastrectomy. Which route should the nurse use to administer cyanocobalamin (vitamin B_{12}) after the surgery?

1. Buccal route
2. Transdermal route
3. Oral route
4. Parenteral route

21. After a nurse teaches a client with diverticular disease about proper diet, he fills out his lunch menu. Which selection by the client demonstrates the need for further teaching?

1. Tossed salad with tomatoes, sunflower seeds, and tuna
2. Egg salad on whole wheat bread and an apple
3. Cottage cheese with apple, pear, and plum slices
4. Ham salad served with whole wheat crackers and a banana

18. 4. A client who avoids conversation about his health may be denying his condition and not coping well with his prognosis. Crying is a normal response to his disease. Asking questions about his prognosis and showing concern for his family are normal coping responses.

CN: Psychological integrity; CNS: None; CL: Analysis

19. 4. Ankylosing spondylitis usually begins between ages 15 to 30 and the prevalence is highest in white males. Back pain is the characteristic feature.

CN: Health promotion and maintenance; CNS: None; CL: Analysis

20. 4. A client who has undergone gastrectomy is no longer able to produce the intrinsic factor necessary for vitamin B_{12} absorption through the GI tract; therefore, the parenteral route (intramuscular or deep subcutaneous injections) is required. This medication isn't available for buccal or transdermal routes.

CN: Physiological integrity; CNS: Pharmacological and parenteral therapies; CL: Application

21. 1. Clients with diverticular disease should avoid high-roughage foods, such as nuts, seeds, popcorn, and raw celery. They should, however, consume high-fiber foods, such as fresh fruit with skins (apples, pears, and plums), bananas, dried fruits, whole wheat bread and crackers, and raw vegetables (lettuce, carrots, and cauliflower).

CN: Physiological integrity; CNS: Basic care and comfort; CL: Application

22. A nurse is teaching nursing students about maintaining a healthy liver. Which measure should the nurse include in her teaching?
1. Take over-the-counter (OTC) medication as needed.
2. Take prescribed medications according to instructions.
3. Add a nutritional supplement to the diet to ensure adequate nutrition.
4. Consume a low-protein diet that contains moderate carbohydrate and fat.

23. A 28-year-old male client complaining of a racing heart and nervousness is admitted to the telemetry floor. His telemetry shows a heart rate of 130 beats/minute in sinus tachycardia. His skin is very warm, dry, and his eyes appear to be bulging. Which nursing action is the most important upon admission?
1. Inserting a urinary catheter and assessing appearance of urine
2. Observing the client's gait
3. Reaching out and feeling the client's neck
4. Standing behind the client and gently palpating the cricothyroid area

24. A client is unemployed, has no health insurance, hasn't filled his levothyroxine (Synthroid) prescription for some time, and has been getting "sicker by the day." Which problem is probably related to him not taking his medication?
1. Diarrhea and vomiting
2. Rapid heart rate
3. Warm, dry, flushed skin
4. Rectal temperature of 94° F (34.4° C)

25. A child with chronic renal failure is scheduled for hemodialysis with an external shunt three times per week. As part of the discharge planning, the nurse should tell the family to perform which step?
1. Assess the site daily for symptoms of redness.
2. Wash the serum at the shunt site with normal saline.
3. Assess the child's blood pressure on the same side as the shunt.
4. Keep a clean dressing in place over the shunt site.

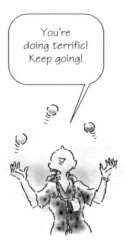

You're doing terrific! Keep going!

22. 2. Taking these measures will help maintain a healthy liver: take prescribed medications according to instructions; avoid taking unnecessary OTC medications; eat a balanced diet that's moderate to high in protein, moderate in carbohydrate and fat, and adequate in vitamins; and take a nutritional supplement only if advised to do so by a physician.
CN: Health promotion and maintenance; CNS: None; CL: Application

23. 4. The client shows signs of hyperthyroidism, and standing behind him and palpating the cricothyroid area is the correct way to assess for an enlarged thyroid gland. Inserting a catheter isn't necessary; assessing the client's urine, which would be concentrated because of dehydration, can be done after he voids. Observing the client's gait isn't necessary at this time.
CN: Physiological integrity; CNS: Physiological adaptation; CL: Analysis

24. 4. Hypothyroidism leads to a hypodynamic state, so a low body temperature is expected after the levothyroxine has been metabolized. Each of the other symptoms is indicative of a hypermetabolic state and, although the client may exhibit these problems, they're probably related to infection and dehydration.
CN: Physiological integrity; CNS: Physiological adaptation; CL: Application

25. 1. The child and parents should assess the shunt site for redness daily because a color change may indicate infection. Serum at the shunt site should be washed away with half strength hydrogen peroxide and an antibiotic ointment applied. Blood pressure shouldn't be taken in the arm with the shunt. A sterile dressing should be placed over the shunt site.
CN: Safe, effective care environment; CNS: Safety and infection control; CL: Application

CN: Client needs category   CNS: Client needs subcategory   CL: Cognitive level

26. A 17-year-old client tells the nurse that she has vulvar itching and a thick, cream-cheese–like vaginal discharge. The nurse anticipates treating the client with which medication?
1. Metronidazole (Flagyl)
2. Erythromycin (Ery-Tab)
3. Miconazole (Monistat)
4. Amoxicillin (Amoxil)

27. When assessing a 5-hour-old neonate, which finding would prompt a nurse to call a physician?
1. Color is dusky, axillary temperature is 96.8° F (37° C), and the baby is spitting up mucus.
2. Hands and feet are cyanotic, abdomen is rounded, and the infant hasn't voided or passed meconium.
3. Anterior fontanel is ¾″ (2 cm) wide, head is molded, and sutures are overriding.
4. Irregular abdominal respirations and intermittent tremors in the extremities.

28. A mother calls the pediatrician because there's an outbreak of scabies at her child's school. The nurse would teach the mother to check for which finding?
1. Pain, erythema, and edema at the site of the bite
2. Oval white dots that adhere to hair shafts
3. Diffuse pruritic wheals
4. Pruritic papules, vesicles, and linear burrows on the finger and toe webs

29. The school nurse assesses a young child with a rash that's raised and has circumscribed areas filled with fluid. The nurse documents this finding as which type of rash?
1. Vesicular rash
2. Papular rash
3. Macular rash
4. Petechial rash

26. 3. The client most likely has *candidiasis,* which produces a thick cream-cheese–like vaginal discharge and is treated with miconazole or nystatin (Mycostatin). Metronidazole is used to treat *Trichomonas vaginalis.* Erythromycin, amoxicillin, or other antibiotic therapy can contribute to *candidiasis* infections and isn't used to treat this infection.
CN: Physiological integrity; CNS: Pharmacological and parenteral therapies; CL: Application

27. 1. Skin color should be pink tinged or ruddy and saliva should be scant. The normal axillary temperature ranges from 97.7° to 98.6° F (36.5° to 37° C). Acrocyanosis may be present for 2 to 6 hours. The neonate should pass meconium and void within 24 hours. Over-riding sutures and molding, when present, may persist for a few days. Neonatal tremors are normal in the neonate; however, they must be evaluated to differentiate them from seizures.
CN: Safe, effective care environment; CNS: Management of care; CL: Application

28. 4. The mother should check her child for pruritic papules, vesicles, and linear burrows on the finger and toe webs. Oval white dots that adhere to the hair shaft can indicate head lice.
CN: Safe, effective care environment; CNS: Safety and infection control; CL: Application

29. 1. A vesicular rash contains small, raised, circumscribed lesions filled with clear fluid. A papular rash contains raised solid lesions with color changes in circumscribed areas. A macular rash is flat with color changes in circumscribed areas. Petechiae are pinpoint purple or red spots on the skin caused by multiple hemorrhages.
CN: Safe, effective care environment; CNS: Safety and infection control; CL: Application

30. A 20-month-old toddler has been treated with permethrin (Nix) for scabies. Because he continues to scratch, his mother wonders whether the drug is working. Which response by a nurse is most appropriate?
   1. "Stop treatment because the drug isn't safe for children under age 2."
   2. "Pruritus can be present for weeks after treatment."
   3. "Apply the drug every day until the rash and itching disappears."
   4. "Pruritus is common in children under age 5 treated with permethrin."

31. An 8-year-old child was sent home after the school reported the presence of head lice. Which information is most helpful to the parents?
   1. The child should remain isolated for 1 week after treatment.
   2. Lindane (Kwell) is the treatment of choice for head lice.
   3. Treatment with a pediculicide followed by combing the hair with a fine-tooth comb will usually kill all lice and remove the nits. Retreatment in 7 to 10 days may be necessary to kill newly hatched lice.
   4. The only way to get rid of head lice is to cut the hair.

32. Which assessment should a nurse do prior to administering disulfiram (Anatabuse) to a client with a history of alcohol abuse?
   1. Assess the client's commitment to attend Alcoholics Anonymous (AA) meetings.
   2. Assess whether the client admits to a problem with alcohol.
   3. Assess when the client's last alcoholic beverage was consumed.
   4. Assess the client's nutritional status.

30. 2. Pruritus may be present for weeks in a child treated with permethrin for scabies. The drug is safe for use in infants as young as age 2 months. Treatment with permethrin can be safely repeated in 2 weeks. Pruritus is caused by secondary reactions of the mites.
CN: Physiological integrity; CNS: Pharmacological and parenteral therapies; CL: Application

31. 3. Treatment with a pediculicide followed by combing the hair with a fine-tooth comb will usually kill all lice and remove the nits. Retreatment in 7 to 10 days may be necessary to kill newly hatched lice. After the infestation has been appropriately treated, there's no reason to isolate the child. Lindane isn't the drug of choice because of its potential for neurotoxicity. The hair should be cut in severe cases only.
CN: Safe, effective care environment; CNS: Safety and infection control; CL: Application

32. 3. The client must be alcohol-free for 12 hours before starting therapy with disulfiram. Assessing the client's commitment to attend AA meetings, the client's perception of his problem, and nutritional status are all important interventions, but they aren't necessary prior to starting disulfiram.
CN: Physiological integrity; CNS: Pharmacological and parenteral therapies; CL: Application

CN: Client needs category   CNS: Client needs subcategory   CL: Cognitive level

33. The nurse is assessing a client with schizophrenia who exhibits negativism, rigidity, excitement, stupor, or posturing. The nurse suspects that the client has which type of schizophrenia?
  1. Catatonic
  2. Undifferentiated
  3. Disorganized
  4. Paranoid

34. Which statement is an example of a key element in a nursing care plan?
  1. Advance diet to regular as tolerated.
  2. Ambulate 30′ (9.1 m) with walker by discharge.
  3. Give furosemide (Lasix) 40 mg I.V. now.
  4. Discontinue I.V. fluids when tolerating oral fluids.

35. A client complains of chronic lower back pain and fatigue and has seen multiple care providers without relief of symptoms. The client insists that something is "terribly wrong." Which action should the nurse take first?
  1. Refer the client for a psychiatric evaluation.
  2. Initiate group therapy for behavior modification.
  3. Obtain a thorough health assessment to rule out physical illnesses.
  4. Refer the client to physical therapy.

36. Which sign alerts a nurse to a possible mild toxic reaction in a client receiving lithium for manic episodes of manic-depressive illness?
  1. Vomiting and diarrhea
  2. Hypertension
  3. Seizures
  4. Increased appetite

33. 1. Catatonic schizophrenia is a state of psychologically induced immobilization, which is, at times, interrupted by episodes of extreme agitation, such as negativism, rigidity, excitement, stupor, or posturing. Undifferentiated schizophrenia occurs when no single clinical presentation dominates (paranoid, disorganized, or catatonic). Disorganized schizophrenia is characterized by disorganized speech, disorganized behavior, and inappropriate affect. The dominant theme in paranoid schizophrenia is one of delusions and hallucinations.
CN: Psychosocial integrity; CNS: None; CL: Application

34. 2. Option 2 is a measurable expected outcome or goal, a key element of a nursing care plan. Other key elements include nursing diagnoses and interventions. The other options are physician's orders, not key elements of nursing care plans.
CN: Safe, effective care environment; CNS: Management of care; CL: Application

35. 3. The first action by the nurse should be to take a thorough health assessment including laboratory studies to rule out physical illnesses. The other actions aren't appropriate until a diagnosis is made.
CN: Safe, effective care environment; CNS: Management of care; CL: Application

36. 1. Vomiting and diarrhea are signs of mild to moderate lithium toxicity. Hypotension, not hypertension, and seizures occur with moderate to severe toxic reactions. Anorexia occurs with mild toxic reactions.
CN: Physiological integrity; CNS: Pharmacological and parenteral therapies; CL: Application

37. A client with bipolar disorder is taking lithium and tells the nurse, "I can stop taking the medicine when I feel better." Which response by the nurse is best?
  1. "That's correct. When you feel better, you can stop taking the medication."
  2. "Take the medication for 1 week after you feel better to be sure there's enough medication in your system."
  3. "Bipolar disorders may require lithium indefinitely to prevent relapses."
  4. "This medication is given as needed. That means that you can take it when you feel that you need it."

38. A client's condition is becoming stabilized after an episode of substance-induced delirium. During the initial recovery period, the nurse should assess the client for which psychosocial health problem?
  1. Flashbacks
  2. Depression
  3. Nightmares
  4. Dissociation

39. A client with a history of depression demonstrates some inconsistent symptoms of cognitive impairment. The nurse should expect which situation when the depression is treated?
  1. Delusional thinking ceases
  2. Recognition of objects improves
  3. Memory problems resolve
  4. Suicidal ideation is no longer a problem

40. A client with borderline personality disorder has extreme views of himself and his situation. Which behavior indicates that the client is a candidate for medication?
  1. Disorientation
  2. Hyperactivity
  3. Regression
  4. Mood swings

You're making great strides!

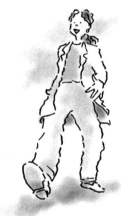

37. 3. Lithium, which helps clients with bipolar disorder stabilize their mood swings, is a long-term treatment. Blood measurements are taken regularly to monitor lithium levels in the client's body. He shouldn't stop taking lithium when he feels better because the therapeutic blood level will decrease. Stopping the medication 1 week after he feels better or taking it as needed will also decrease the therapeutic blood level of lithium.

CN: Physiological integrity; CNS: Pharmacological and parenteral therapies; CL: Analysis

38. 2. Depression and anxiety are common mental health problems seen immediately after substance withdrawal. Flashbacks and nightmares are commonly observed in clients with posttraumatic stress disorder. Dissociation occurs when a client undergoes prolonged physical and sexual abuse.

CN: Psychosocial integrity; CNS: None; CL: Analysis

39. 3. In a condition called *pseudodementia,* a client treated for depression will have a dramatic improvement in memory. Delusional thinking and object-recognition problems aren't characteristic of pseudodementia. The nurse must assess all clients with depression for suicidal ideation because they're at some degree of risk for suicide.

CN: Psychosocial integrity; CNS: None; CL: Application

40. 4. Medications aren't typically given to clients with personality disorders. However, clients with mood swings, hallucinations, or psychotic behaviors are appropriate candidates for medications. Disorientation, hyperactivity and regression aren't necessarily seen in clients with borderline personality disorders.

CN: Psychosocial integrity; CNS: None; CL: Application

CN: Client needs category   CNS: Client needs subcategory   CL: Cognitive level

41. A client has traits of an avoidant personality disorder. Which family intervention should the nurse give the highest priority in the care plan?
1. Explaining that the family should teach the client social skills.
2. Recommending that the family recognize the client's high sensitivity to criticism.
3. Exploring ways for the family to help the client express true feelings.
4. Asking the family to keep a daily log of the client's adjustment difficulties.

42. A client with a substance abuse disorder says the problem doesn't really exist. Which intervention should be the nurse's initial one?
1. Educating about the principles of mental health
2. Examining the use of defense mechanisms
3. Recognizing and discussing feelings of resentment
4. Discussing the need for a caretaker while in recovery

43. A nurse is evaluating drug therapy effectiveness in a client undergoing alcohol detoxification. Which finding indicates that drug therapy needs to be adjusted?
1. There are signs of toxicity from the drug.
2. The drug prevents the occurrence of further problems.
3. During the course of treatment, the dosage has increased.
4. The drug facilitates the client's interactions with staff.

44. A nurse explains the unit's rules to a client with bulimia nervosa. Which action by the client indicates that learning has occurred?
1. The client asks to be accompanied to the bathroom after lunch.
2. The client writes down every food item eaten in the past 24 hours.
3. The client decides to help the dietitian plan the unit's meals.
4. The client discusses current problems with the nurse before mealtime.

41. 2. A client with traits of an avoidant personality disorder is very sensitive to criticism and disapproval but doesn't typically have learning or social skills problems. Such a client may have difficulty expressing feelings and may have few friends or only family members for interaction. Having the family keep a log of the client's adjustment difficulties isn't an appropriate intervention; the list may be interpreted as a statement of rejection.
CN: Safe, effective care environment; CNS: Management of care; CL: Analysis

42. 2. Defense mechanisms contribute to the client's denial. Education won't be well received unless the client recognizes the problem and determines that the nurse's teaching would be useful. The client can't recognize and discuss feelings of resentment when denying that a problem exists. The client needs to become responsible for his own behavior and take care of himself.
CN: Psychosocial integrity; CNS: None; CL: Application

43. 1. If signs of toxicity from drug therapy occur during the detoxification period, the drug therapy needs to be adjusted. The medication is working if it prevents further problems. Sometimes, the dosage must be adjusted to obtain the maximum benefit. If the drug enables the client to have therapeutic interactions with the staff, the client is benefiting from the therapy.
CN: Physiological integrity; CNS: Pharmacological and parenteral therapies; CL: Application

44. 1. When the client asks to be accompanied to the bathroom after a meal, the client is following protocol for restoring healthy eating and promoting adequate nutrition. This action indicates the client's commitment to not purging after a meal. Recording the food eaten in a 24-hour period would be appropriate for a client with anorexia nervosa, not a client with bulimia nervosa. It's inappropriate for a client to plan meals for the unit's clients. The client can discuss problems any time, not just before mealtimes.
CN: Psychosocial integrity; CNS: None; CL: Analysis

45. A nurse is teaching a client with an eating disorder about cues that trigger unhealthy eating behaviors. Which example explains social cues?
  1. Diet advertisements
  2. Troublesome memories
  3. Interpersonal conflict
  4. Frustration fatigue

46. A schizophrenic client states, "The voices keep talking to me. They're telling me that I have to leave here and that I shouldn't talk to you. Don't you hear what they're saying?" Which response is best?
  1. "You didn't take your medicine this morning, did you?"
  2. "The voices aren't real. You're sick and they're part of your illness."
  3. "Are you hearing voices again?"
  4. " I don't hear the voices, but I see that you are upset."

47. The nurse is teaching caregivers about the signs and symptoms of schizophrenia relapse. Which response by the caregivers about the signs and symptoms to report to a mental health professional indicates that the teaching has been effective?
  1. Changes in appetite resulting in weight loss or gain
  2. Loss of interest in sexual activities
  3. Increased socialization
  4. Feelings of tenseness and difficulty sleeping

48. A client with schizophrenia has been prescribed risperidone (Risperdal). The client's symptoms include hallucinations, delusions, and withdrawal. A nurse explains that the medication will help improve which symptoms?
  1. Negative symptoms
  2. Positive symptoms
  3. Negative and positive symptoms
  4. Paranoid symptoms

45. 3. Social cues that trigger maladaptive behavior include feelings of isolation and conflict with family or friends. Diet advertisements are considered situational cues. Troublesome memories are psychological cues. Frustration fatigue is an example of a physiological cue.
CN: Psychosocial integrity; CNS: None; CL: Application

46. 4. The nurse should be honest and tell the client that she doesn't hear the voices while acknowledging the client's feelings. Asking if the client took his medication or explaining his illness doesn't allow the client to feel valued by the nurse. Asking him if he hears voices makes him feel that the nurse wasn't listening.
CN: Psychosocial integrity; CNS: None; CL: Application

47. 4. Signs and symptoms of schizophrenia relapse include difficulty concentrating and sleeping, feelings of tenseness, and increased bizarre thinking and withdrawal. The other choices aren't signs and symptoms of schizophrenia.
CN: Psychosocial integrity; CNS: None; CL: Analysis

48. 3. Risperidone targets both negative and positive symptoms. Positive symptoms include delusions, hallucinations, and bizarre behaviors. Negative symptoms indicate a loss or lack of normal functioning such as lack of motivation and social withdrawal.
CN: Physiological integrity; CNS: Pharmacological and parenteral therapies; CL: Application

CN: Client needs category   CNS: Client needs subcategory   CL: Cognitive level

49. A newly graduated nurse is caring for a client recently diagnosed with dissociative identity disorder. The nurse asks the preceptor about discussing a client's traumatic childhood with the client. Which advice from the preceptor is best?
1. "Ask pointed questions and demand specific answers."
2. "If the client begins talking about it, just listen and be supportive."
3. "Tell the client that you suspect that much of his memory is exaggerated."
4. "Tell the client that those issues can be discussed with a physician only."

50. A client with dissociative identity disorder frequently switches from one personality to another. The nurse can identify the switch by which finding?
1. Episodes of orthostatic hypotension
2. Blinking or rolling the eyes frequently
3. Dystonic reactions
4. Episodes of tachycardia

51. A 38-year-old female client is scheduled to have a hysterectomy and is concerned about no longer being a "whole woman." Which intervention by the nurse is best?
1. Tell her to talk to her husband about the permanent changes that will be taking place with her body.
2. Refer her to group therapy.
3. Encourage her to discuss her concerns and feelings.
4. Give her information to read and leave the room.

52. A 23-year-old female client is seen in the emergency department for rape. The woman is very calm and appears emotionally unaffected by the event. Which assessment of the client's behavior is appropriate?
1. The client probably isn't telling the truth but is trying to get the perpetrator in trouble.
2. The client was a willing partner.
3. The client's initially deceptive calm may be masking distress, denial, or emotional shock.
4. The client is pregnant and is trying to blame the pregnancy on a rape.

49. 2. If the subject is painful, the client will discuss it when he feels comfortable and ready. Forcing him to talk about the subject will cause severe anxiety and result in distrust. The other choices don't facilitate a trusting relationship between the nurse and the client.
CN: Safe, effective care environment; CNS: Management of care; CL: Application

50. 2. Switching from one personality to another is manifested in a number of ways including blinking, facial movements, and changes in voice. Changes in blood pressure or pulse or dystonic reactions aren't indicative of switching from one personality to another.
CN: Psychosocial integrity; CNS: None; CL: Application

51. 3. The nurse should encourage the client to express her feelings. Telling her to talk to her husband will cause the client added concern and anxiety. Referring her to group therapy isn't an appropriate intervention at this time. Giving her information and leaving the room doesn't allow her to ask questions and express concerns.
CN: Psychosocial integrity; CNS: None; CL: Analysis

52. 3. One of the immediate consequences of rape is deceptive calmness. This behavior usually masks emotional shock, denial, or distress. The other responses are judgmental opinions. Nurses are to remain nonjudgmental in providing care.
CN: Psychosocial integrity; CNS: None; CL: Analysis

53. A full-term neonate was just admitted to the transitional nursery. He has a large meningomyelocele covered by an intact sac. The nurse knows immediately to place this neonate on his stomach with hips slightly elevated. Which statement describes the rationale for this position?
   1. To prevent the sac covering the defect from rupturing
   2. To preserve urine and bowel control
   3. To assess neurologic functioning more easily
   4. To prevent further neurologic damage

54. A nurse is teaching the mother of a neonate with a cleft palate how to feed him. Which instruction should the nurse give the mother?
   1. Feed the neonate in a semi-reclining position with his head resting on the mother's curved elbow.
   2. Feed the neonate in an upright position.
   3. Feed the neonate lying on his stomach with his head turned toward his mother.
   4. Feed the neonate in any position that the mother and child are comfortable.

55. A nurse observes school-age children playing. Which activity is typical of this age-group?
   1. Barbie dolls
   2. Monopoly
   3. Sony Play Station video games
   4. Hot Wheels cars

56. A nurse is assessing an infant's growth and development. Which action by the nurse indicates the best understanding of a 4-month-old's stage of growth and development?
   1. Eliciting a social smile
   2. Allowing the infant to hold his own bottle
   3. Playing peek-a-boo with the infant
   4. Letting the infant sit without support

Keep moving along! You're almost finished!

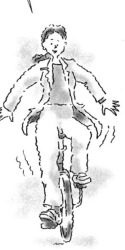

53. 1. The sac covering the defect is the only barrier preventing bacteria from directly entering the neonate's central nervous system and causing meningitis and encephalitis. A large defect will result in loss of urine and bowel control. The nurse can assess neurologic functioning when the child is on his back or stomach. The damage to the neurologic system happened in utero, and the nurse should prevent further damage by placing the infant on his stomach until after surgery. Preventing neurologic damage isn't the priority.
CN: Physiological integrity; CNS: Reduction of risk potential; CL: Analysis

54. 2. Feed the neonate with a cleft palate in an upright position. Incorrect feeding can allow formula to slip through the palate opening, enter the upper respiratory tract and lungs, and cause aspiration pneumonia. Any of the other positions is placing the neonate at risk for aspiration pneumonia.
CN: Physiological integrity; CNS: Reduction of risk potential; CL: Analysis

55. 2. School-age children engage in competitive play with established rules and goals. Monopoly is an excellent example of play that pulls these elements together. Playing with Barbie dolls is an example of associative play, which preschoolers engage in. Solitary play of video games is seen in adolescents. Playing with Hot Wheels cars is more indicative of toddlers' parallel play.
CN: Health promotion and maintenance; CNS: None; CL: Application

56. 1. A social smile should be seen in a 4-month-old. An infant can't hold his own bottle until age 6 to 7 months, and he'll engage in peek-a-boo activity at age 10 to 12 months. He can sit without support at about age 8 months.
CN: Health promotion and maintenance; CNS: None; CL: Application

CN: Client needs category   CNS: Client needs subcategory   CL: Cognitive level

57. The nurse is caring for an 11-year-old client with cerebral palsy who has a pressure ulcer on the sacrum. When teaching the client's mother about dietary intake, which foods should the nurse plan to emphasize?
1. Legumes and cheese
2. Whole grain products
3. Fruits and vegetables
4. Lean meats and low fat milk

57. 4. Although the client should eat a balanced diet with foods from all food groups, the diet should emphasize foods that supply complete protein, such as lean meats and low-fat milk. Protein helps build and repair body tissue, which promotes healing. Legumes provide incomplete protein. Cheese contains complete protein but also fat, which should be limited to 30% or less of caloric intake. Whole grain products supply incomplete proteins and carbohydrates. Fruits and vegetables mainly provide carbohydrates.
CN: Physiological integrity; CNS: Basic care and comfort; CL: Application

58. A client is diagnosed with pneumonia. Which nursing diagnosis would take priority for this client?
1. *Excess fluid volume*
2. *Ineffective airway clearance*
3. *Activity intolerance*
4. *Deficient knowledge*

58. 2. Pneumonia refers to inflammation of the lungs, and can produce copious amounts of tracheobronchial secretions. These secretions interfere with airway patency and gas exchange. Therefore, airway clearance is a priority. The client may experience a decrease in fluid volume, not an excess, due to increased temperature and respiratory rate. The client also may experience activity intolerance and deficient knowledge, but neither is the priority diagnosis.
CN: Safe, effective care environment: CNS: Management of care; CL: Analysis

59. A nurse is caring for a client in active labor. Which observation would cause the nurse to suspect fetal distress?
1. Fetal heart rate of 144 beats/minute
2. Accelerations of the fetal heart rate with contractions
3. Fetal scalp pH of 7.14
4. Presence of long-term variability

59. 3. A scalp pH below 7.25 indicates acidosis and fetal hypoxia. A fetal heart rate of 144 beats/ minute, acceleration of the fetal heartbeat with contractions, and the presence of long-term variability with contractions are normal responses of a healthy fetus to labor.
CN: Health promotion and maintenance; CNS: None; CL: Application

60. During a routine examination, the mother of a 3-month-old child asks the nurse, "How soon will she have her first tooth?" Which response by the nurse would be the most accurate as to the age by which the first tooth usually erupts?
1. 4 months
2. 5 months
3. 6 months
4. 7 months

60. 3. The first tooth typically erupts at age 6 months, although some infants do get their first tooth when a little younger or older.
CN: Health promotion and maintenance; CNS: None; CL: Application

61. A nurse assesses an 18-month-old toddler. Which activity would indicate to the nurse that the child is exhibiting normal growth and development patterns?
1. Running and jumping in place
2. Jumping down from a chair
3. Naming a specific color
4. Saying his full name

61. 1. An 18-month-old child should be able to run and jump in place. Typically, a child of 30 months is able to jump down from a chair, can name one color, and knows his full name.
CN: Health promotion and maintenance; CNS: None; CL: Application

62. A mother was diagnosed with polyhydramnios during her pregnancy and just delivered a preterm male neonate. In which manner should the nurse assess a neonate for tracheoesophageal fistula?
1. Observing the neonate during the first formula feeding
2. Determining if cyanosis is present at birth
3. Inserting a catheter through the esophagus to the stomach
4. Assessing lung sounds to determine if possible pneumonia is present

63. Which instruction should be included in the care plan for a client following total hip replacement?
1. Keeping the legs adducted
2. Not bending at the hip more than 90 degrees
3. Keeping the hips lower than the knees when seated
4. Teaching how to bend forward to put on socks and shoes

64. Which cause of myocarditis is the most common?
1. Bacteria
2. Parasite
3. Fungus
4. Virus

62. 3. Tracheoesophageal fistula is present if a catheter can't be passed through the neonate's esophagus to the stomach. A barium swallow or a bronchial endoscopy examination will reveal the blind-end esophagus. The condition should be diagnosed before the infant is fed; otherwise, the infant will cough and may become cyanotic during feeding. Immediately after birth, pneumonia shouldn't be present with a tracheoesophageal fistula. Emergency surgery is essential to prevent pneumonia caused by the stomach's contents leaking into the lungs.
CN: Health promotion and maintenance; CNS: None; CL: Analysis

63. 2. Following a total hip replacement, the client should be instructed not to bend more than 90 degrees at the hip. The legs should be kept abducted to prevent dislocation of the prosthesis. The hips should be kept higher than the knees when seated to minimize hip flexion. The client should be instructed not to bend forward at the hip to put on shoes and socks. Assistive devices can be used to help the client safely dress below the waist.
CN: Physiological integrity; CNS: Reduction of risk potential; CL: Application

64. 4. Myocarditis (inflammation of the myocardium) is usually caused by a virus. Of all the viruses, coxsackieviruses and echoviruses are the most common agents. Bacteria, parasites, and fungi may cause myocarditis, but they aren't the most common causes.
CN: Physiological integrity; CNS: Physiological adaptation; CL: Analysis

CN: Client needs category   CNS: Client needs subcategory   CL: Cognitive level

65. A nurse is caring for a 7-year-old client receiving cyclophosphamide (Cytoxan). In addition to administering mesna (Mesnex), which action should the nurse take?
1. Transfusing platelets before administering the drug
2. Giving the child cranberry juice to drink
3. Encouraging the child to void frequently
4. Limiting the child's fluid intake

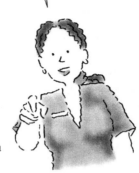

Only 10 more questions. Can you believe it?

66. When protective isolation isn't indicated, a nurse plans which activity for a child receiving chemotherapy?
1. Bed rest
2. Activity as tolerated
3. Walk to bathroom only
4. Out of bed for brief periods

67. A child is intubated and placed on a ventilator after a near drowning. The physician's order is to suction every 3 to 4 hours. The child's parents ask the nurse why the suctioning is necessary. Which response by the nurse is the most accurate?
1. To keep the client free of infection
2. To keep the client from experiencing cardiac arrhythmias
3. To keep the client's airway patent
4. To maintain fluid and electrolyte balance

68. A child with cystic fibrosis has a bronchodilator, steroids ordered by metered-dose inhaler, and chest physiotherapy. In which order should these medications and treatments be administered?
1. Perform chest physiotherapy first.
2. Administer the bronchodilator first.
3. Administer the steroid first.
4. Let the client eat lunch first and then perform chest physiotherapy.

65. 3. Hemorrhagic cystitis can result when the by-products of cyclophosphamide metabolism remain in the bladder; therefore, emptying the bladder at least every 2 hours when the child is awake can help prevent this painful condition. The child should be encouraged to void as soon as the urge is felt. Bacteria or low platelets don't cause the condition, so transfusing platelets and giving cranberry juice aren't correct. Limiting fluid is contraindicated. Instead, the child will be given fluids liberally, usually by I.V. infusion, and encouraged to drink; a high intake of fluids will increase elimination of the drug's toxic by-products.
CN: Physiological integrity; CNS: Pharmacological and parenteral therapies; CL: Analysis

66. 2. Children receiving chemotherapy should be able to engage in activities of interest and maintain as much independence and autonomy as possible; they'll limit their activity when they feel tired or ill. Limiting their activities to bed rest, walking to bathroom only, or only out of bed for brief periods isn't necessary and restricts activity unnecessarily. Whenever possible, include children in planning their care. These children should avoid adults and other children with infections.
CN: Health promotion and maintenance; CNS: None; CL: Application

67. 3. Because of the increased secretions from drowning, the airway is more prone to obstruction, and suctioning is essential for maintaining patency. Suctioning won't prevent infection and may even cause it. Suctioning can cause bradycardia; therefore, preoxygenation is essential to prevent arrhythmias. Suctioning doesn't affect fluid and electrolyte balance.
CN: Physiological integrity; CNS: Reduction of risk potential; CL: Application

68. 2. Administer the bronchodilator to dilate the bronchi. The steroid can then reach further down the respiratory tract. After each medication is given, perform chest physiotherapy to expectorate secretions in the lower airways. Administer the medications and chest physiotherapy before meals to prevent aspiration.
CN: Physiological integrity; CNS: Pharmacological and parental therapies; CL: Application

69. A nurse is teaching a student nurse about ketogenic diet. Which condition would the nurse state is a ketogenic diet sometimes used to treat?
1. Anorexia nervosa
2. Nephrotic syndrome
3. Epilepsy
4. Ulcerative colitis

70. A child is unable to walk without assistance because of decreased oxygen at birth. Which disorder is characterized by a malfunction of the brain's motor center from hypoxia?
1. Down syndrome
2. Cerebral palsy
3. Sickle cell anemia
4. Osteogenesis imperfecta

71. A 17-year-old client who injured his right knee during a basketball game is scheduled for an arthroscopy. The nurse teaches the client about the procedure. Which response by the nurse regarding arthroscopy would be accurate?
1. An X-ray using a contrast media
2. Visualization of the joint with a small instrument
3. Inserting a needle and withdrawing fluid for biopsy
4. Aspirating synovial fluid from the bursa

72. A nurse is assessing a 13-year-old child 12 hours after surgery for a compound-fracture repair of the right arm. Which finding requires immediate attention?
1. Bruising of the fingers
2. Capillary refill of 3 seconds
3. Pallor of the nail beds
4. Edema of the extremity

69. 3. A ketogenic diet is typically suggested as a method of treatment for epilepsy. Anorexia nervosa is treated with counseling and slowly reintroducing food. Children with nephrotic syndrome are usually on a low-sodium diet. Ulcerative colitis is treated with a low-residue diet.
CN: Physiological integrity; CNS: Reduction of risk potential; CL: Application

70. 2. Cerebral palsy affects the motor center of the brain and is usually caused by brain trauma. Down syndrome is a chromosomal abnormality. Sickle cell anemia is a genetic disorder of red blood cells. Osteogenesis imperfecta is a congenital anomaly involving decreased calcium in the bones and leads to multiple fractures at birth.
CN: Physiological integrity; CNS: Physiological adaptation; CL: Application

71. 2. After a small incision is made in the knee, a small tube-shaped instrument is inserted for viewing the knee and surrounding cartilage, tendon, and ligaments. Contrast media is typically used for X-rays of joints. Biopsies are taken if cancer is a concern. Synovial fluid is collected for culture if an infection or inflammation is a concern.
CN: Physiological integrity; CNS: Physiological adaptation; CL: Application

72. 3. Pallor suggests a decrease in circulation to the extremity, and the surgeon should be notified. Bruising can be expected with a compound fracture. The fingers should be observed for further discoloration indicating decreased circulation. Capillary refill of 3 seconds is normal. Edema is expected but should be watched; increased edema might impair circulation.
CN: Physiological integrity; CNS: Reduction of risk potential; CL: Application

CN: Client needs category   CNS: Client needs subcategory   CL: Cognitive level

73. A 3-year-old child has diarrhea, and the pediatrician has recommended a BRAT diet for the next 24 hours. The nurse teaches the parents about the diet. Which response by the parents about the diet indicates the teaching has been effective? "The diet consists of:
1. bran, rice crispies, apple juice, and tomato juice."
2. beans, red meat, apples, and tomatoes."
3. bananas, rice, applesauce, and toast."
4. broccoli, red ice pops, apple butter, and tacos."

74. After undergoing small-bowel resection, a client is prescribed metronidazole (Flagyl) 500 mg I.V. The mixed I.V. solution contains 100 ml. A nurse is to run the drug over 30 minutes. The drip factor of the available I.V. tubing is 15 gtt/ml. What is the drip rate? Record your answer usng a whole number.

_____ gtt/minute

75. A nurse is caring for a client whose cultural background is different from her own. Which actions are appropriate? Select all that apply:
1. Consider that nonverbal cues, such as eye contact, may have different meanings in different cultures.
2. Respect the client's cultural beliefs.
3. Ask the client if he has cultural or religious requirements that should be considered in his care.
4. Explain your beliefs so that the client will understand the differences.
5. Understand that all cultures experience pain in the same way.

73. 3. BRAT stands for bananas, rice, applesauce, and toast. This diet is commonly used for children with diarrhea because these foods add some form to the stool without further irritating the bowel. The other diet choices can cause gas, irritation, and inflammation in the already inflamed bowel.
CN: Physiological integrity; CNS: Basic care and comfort; CL: Application

74. 50. Use the following equation: 100 ml/30 minutes × 15 gtt/1 ml = 49.9 gtt/minute (50 gtt/minute).
CN: Physiological integrity; CNS: Pharmacological and parenteral therapies; CL: Application

75. 1, 2, 3. Nonverbal cues may have different meanings in different cultures. In one culture, eye contact is a sign of disrespect; in another, eye contact shows respect and attentiveness. The nurse should always respect the client's cultural beliefs and ask if he has cultural or religious requirements. This may include food choices or restrictions, body coverings, or time for prayer. The nurse should attempt to understand the client's culture; it isn't the client's responsibility to understand the nurse's culture. The nurse should never impose her own beliefs on her clients. Culture influences a client's experience of pain. For example, in one culture pain may be openly expressed, whereas in another culture it may be quietly endured.
CN: Psychosocial integrity; CNS: None; CL: Analysis

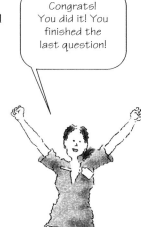

Congrats! You did it! You finished the last question!

DATE DUE